A Global History of Child Death

PETER LANG
New York • Bern • Frankfurt • Berlin
Brussels • Vienna • Oxford • Warsaw

AMY J. CATALANO

A Global History of Child Death

MORTALITY, BURIAL, AND PARENTAL ATTITUDES

PETER LANG
New York • Bern • Frankfurt • Berlin
Brussels • Vienna • Oxford • Warsaw

Library of Congress Cataloging-in-Publication Data

Catalano, Amy J.
A global history of child death: mortality, burial,
and parental attitudes / Amy J. Catalano.
pages cm
Includes bibliographical references and index.
1. Children—Mortality—History. 2. Children—Death—History.
3. Burial—History. 4. Mourning customs—History. I. Title.
HB1323.C5C37 304.6'4083—dc23 2014014814
ISBN 978-1-4331-2742-7 (hardcover)
ISBN 978-1-4539-1361-1 (e-book)

Bibliographic information published by **Die Deutsche Nationalbibliothek.**
Die Deutsche Nationalbibliothek lists this publication in the "Deutsche Nationalbibliografie"; detailed bibliographic data are available on the Internet at http://dnb.d-nb.de/.

Cover image: Joshua Reynolds, Sketch of Putto
Holding a Sash in Both Hands, Seen from Below

The paper in this book meets the guidelines for permanence and durability of the Committee on Production Guidelines for Book Longevity of the Council of Library Resources.

29 Broadway, 18th floor, New York, NY 10006
www.peterlang.com

Printed in Germany

For Sophia, Luciano, Grace, and Lilly…

"It's so mysterious, the land of tears."

The Little Prince by Antoine de Saint-Exupéry

Contents

Acknowledgments

To my colleague Gloria Grant Roberson for the title, and for encouraging me to continue writing and researching. To my colleagues at Hofstra University in both the library and the School of Education for their support and kindness. To Lynne Catalano, Tony Catalano, Emily Schwartz, and Sophia Cianciulli who read various drafts of this work and provided valuable input. To my husband Jon for helping with the children and housework so that I could take time to work on this book. To Dr. Ben Potter who graciously offered me advice on terminology and earlier drafts of Chapter 2. To the chair of my department, Georgina Martorella, for her enthusiastic support.

Credit is due to the following for allowing me to reprint portions of poems:

Aaron Kramer, *The Last Lullaby: Poetry from the Holocaust* (Syracuse: Syracuse University Press, 1997), 34, 39. © SUP. Reproduced with Permission from the Publisher.

Barbara Crooker, *The Lost Children* (1984), Reproduced with Permission from the Author.

Introduction

Parental Attitudes toward Children

When Aries proposed that in cultures and historical eras where a large percentage of children did not live to see their first or second birthday, parents were often indifferent to the death of a child. He states that this is an "inevitable direct consequence of the demographic situation of that time".[1] Some researchers examining familial histories have come to a similar conclusion. Yet in the last thirty years others have come to criticize this view, which at times has been based on selective data, as well as interpretations based on modern views of parent-child relationships.[2] Evidence of parental attitudes toward their children is vast and diverse. For example, diaries of colonial Americans reveal deep affection for one's children, while other evidence appears to reflect ambivalence. The widespread practice of infanticide from prehistory to the present is also indicative of the complexity of parental grief and concern.

This book aims to examine the culture of parent-child relationships, and more specifically parental concern for the child, by investigating the mortuary behavior associated with a child's death. The scope of this book is global. Funerary behavior is observed from the Prehistoric to Modern era. The thesis of this book is not to claim that parental grief over a child's death indicates parental concern. Rather, I seek to provide a layered perspective of the complex feelings parents demonstrated toward their children in different cultures, in different historical eras, and through particular situations within those time periods. Parental concern has been examined by many historians and a brief review of this research is discussed here. It provides us with a context within which to place views of child death.

Aries' view of children in the medieval period may be explained by the perception that children were considered to be "little adults", a view in contention with more recent research.[3] He asserts that children were "mixed in" with adults as soon as they could fare without their caregivers—around the age of seven. Aries also claims that there was no recognized period for childhood and adolescence because there were no words for it.[4] Children, however, had toys and play was their first profession. Childhood, and all that goes with it, *was* recognized as a stage in the "life of man" and it may be inferred, nurtured. Children were protected and mourned when they died, even those that were unknown. Barbara Hanawalt counters the assumption that there was general callousness toward a child's death in medieval London, for example, with evidence to the contrary. In some cases, dead children abandoned in a London church were offered a proper burial by wealthy members of the church.[5] Perhaps impoverished parents anticipated this generosity in their act of desertion.

While Aries' thesis focuses on the Middle Ages in France, it is generalized toward the entire West. More recently, Shorter claims "'Good mothering is an invention of modernization'...children were held in such low esteem that they were not even regarded as human...' Nor did these mothers often see their infants as human beings with the same capacities for joy and pain- as they themselves'".[6] We will find that this claim is absurd given the opposing evidence in many societies throughout history. While one may infer that these attitudes toward children, supported by Aries and Shorter, were indicative of only societies where child mortality rates were high, child and infant mortality has been elevated up until the conventions of modern medicine in the industrialized world. In fact, Pollock asserts that the high rate of infant mortality increased anxiety over a child's death rather than facilitated ambivalence.[7]

McLaughlin and Lyman both counter Aries' claims that there was no appreciation of childhood. Lyman believes that "up till the 8th century parents were ambivalent towards their offspring, viewing them both as a pleasure and an integral part of family life, as well as a 'bother'." The latter was more often the standard perspective. McLaughlin, studying children from the 9th to 13th centuries, claimed that there were "clear signs of tenderness toward infants and small children... [and] awareness of their need for love".[8]

The evidence of ill-treatment of children is copious. Grief demonstrated by a parent over the death of his or her child did not necessarily reflect love for the child while alive. Morelli, in admonishment to the parent who grieves over the death of child, says "You loved him but never used your love to make him happy; you treated him more like a stranger than a son; you never gave him an hour of rest…You never kissed him when he wanted it; you wore him out at school and with many harsh blows".[9] deMause explains that it is not love that parents lacked for their children, but emotional maturity to see that children did not exist to project the needs of the parent.[10]

Pollock, among other historians, notes that grief over the death of an older child is far greater than that for an infant. It appears that while parental distress over the death of an infant was often expressed, many parents resigned themselves to the fact that most children would ultimately die in infancy. Slater, in his study of child death in the Puritan era (New England, 1620–1720) states that "parental apprehensiveness about death had a different quality [than that of modern society]. Mothers and fathers genuinely expected to lose some of their babies. The Puritans saw infants passing away at a disheartening rate, fragile, death-prone beings."[11] In the Puritan era, one of every ten infants died, whereas presently in the United States six infants (under the age of 1) die for every 1000 live births.[12] Further, while parents of any era may grieve copiously at the first child death, they may exhibit more steadfastness in the presence of other deaths.

Some historians have also failed to consider the different causes of seemingly negligent behavior toward a child by a parent as a product of social class. For example, a medieval peasant mother who leaves her children dirty may be deemed a careless parent. However, such actions, interpreted through the lens of farming society in the Middle Ages, may be read as an attempt to keep malevolent spirits from the child and thus death.[13] Conversely, poor women who had to work may have had no other option but to leave their infants and children alone or bring them to work. In one case, a medieval woman brought her child to work only to have it beaten so severely by the apprentice that it died two days later.[14]

Another often misunderstood indicator of ambivalence toward children is the lack of burial rites for infants. Rawson states that reasons for the absence of memorialization for infants under one or two years old is that in "most, perhaps all, societies, a child is not considered a 'real' person until it has developed certain functions" such as the ability to walk or speak.[15] The high rate of neonatal deaths in ancient and medieval societies, as well as in modern third world countries, is often cast as a reason for emotional distance from infants. This theme is peddled over and over again by historians; however, more recent research on infant death in high mortality societies indicates that grief over the deaths of the very young is very real.[16]

It is important to remember that the evidence left us by the artifacts of death does not always provide an accurate window into the inner emotions or even the behavior of the bereaved. Cultural expectations often persuade the grieving to betray their emotions in favor of pride, self-restraint and dignity. For example, Gil'adi discusses the expectation of medieval Muslim parents to withhold their grief publicly despite other evidence left to us in the consolation literature during that period.[17] The steadfastness demonstrated by medieval parents was often misunderstood. Because of these cultural and societal miscommunications, in his study of consolation treatises, written during the height of the Black Death for parents of young children, Gil'adi disputes Aries' claim of parental indifference toward the deaths of children.[18]

Interestingly, mourning among the upper class Romans was said to be staid in the interest of self-restraint. Aristocrats, though, also had avenues within which to express their grief, such as consolatory literature and funeral rituals, whereas those from the lower classes did not have access to these vehicles of expression, and therefore grieved more openly and uninhibitedly.[19]

Childhood historians appear to agree that the high rates of child death led to the neglect of children, and therefore, even higher rates of mortality.[20] Stone and others argue that in order to preserve their mental stability, parents were obliged to limit the degree of emotional involvement with their infant children. "Ephemeral" is the word Stone uses to describe infants in early modern England.[21] Surely this perspective of infant life would have bred neglect and a self-perpetuating circle of death. On the other hand, "When infant deaths are frequent, it is argued, infant survival becomes a high-priority parental goal".[22]

Van Setten discusses the shift in Dutch parents' attention toward child death in the seventeenth through nineteenth centuries. Parents appeared to grieve more openly in the latter century. While his discussion focuses on photographs and consolatory literature, Van Setten asks the pertinent question: "Why the change in attitude?" Demographic evidence of this time suggests that the change is related to the lower death rate of children, although he argues that it is truly a change in mentality. Most notably, the bourgeois family ideal which "aimed at conscious cultivation of emotional relations" indicated a shift toward the sentimental.[23] Conversely, some family historians contend that reactions of parents toward their dead children do not necessarily indicate loving attitudes. deMause has noted that "Expressions of tenderness toward children occur most often when the child is non-demanding, especially when the child is either asleep or dead."[24]

In what follows, parental attitudes are examined across cultures and through time. It is important to remember that historical attitudes should not be viewed through the lens of modern expectations.[25] Attitudes toward children are complex phenomena shaped by historical circumstances and cultural values at the very least. By examining mortuary behaviors within the wide lens of history, literature, art, archaeology and science we can put cultural practices into context.

This book is organized into two parts. Part one begins with an overview of child mortality; its causes, prevention, and extent through time, followed by an exploration of the ways in which children were buried and mourned, and sometimes killed by their parents, from prehistory through the early modern era. Part Two examines other indicators of parental attitudes toward child death; consolation literature, artwork and photography, naming practices, and replacement, as well as infanticide and child sacrifice.

Part I

Mortality and Burial Practices through History

1 A Brief History of Child Mortality

Infancy, like old age, was a time to die.[1]

Before investigating the sociological and psychological reactions of a society, and specifically parents, to the death of a child, it is helpful to frame the discussion within the matter of actual mortality among regions across time. This chapter gives an overview of conditions that existed during times, and in places, where child mortality was particularly high. This chapter does not seek to provide a complete history of child mortality. Throughout this book wherever possible I provide mortality rates, but these numbers should be accepted with caution as they can drastically change in one country within just a few decades. Social and political changes often facilitate the decrease of mortality rates and these efforts will also be discussed.

Achieving one's fifth birthday is an extraordinary milestone in many developing countries, and is usually indicative of a life that is likely to mature to a healthy adulthood. In fact, according to the World Health Organization (WHO), the mortality of children under the age of five is the leading indicator of overall health and development of countries. At the United Nations' 2000 Millennium Summit, 189 world leaders committed themselves to ending "extreme poverty" by 2015 by addressing eight specific Goals.[2] Millennium Goal 4 calls for reducing the under-five mortality rate by two thirds between 1990 and 2015.

The United Nations Inter-agency Group notes that substantial progress has been made towards Goal 4 in that mortality of children under the age of five dropped thirty-five percent from 1990 to 2010. Nevertheless, 6.6 million children under the age of five perished in 2012, and forty-five percent of these deaths were attributed to malnutrition.

The highest rates of child mortality exist in Sub-Saharan Africa where one of every eight children dies before the age of five, and in Southern Asia where the rate is one in fifteen. In developed nations the mortality rate for children under the age of five is one in every 143, and is acutely declining, contributing to an ever widening disparity between Sub-Saharan Africa and Southern Asia and the rest of the world. Fifty percent of under-five deaths are concentrated in India, Nigeria, Democratic Republic of the Congo, Pakistan and China. India and Nigeria account for thirty-three percent of these deaths.

While the majority of under-five deaths occur within the first year of life, the first month of life (the neonatal period) is the most vulnerable. Thirty percent of neonatal deaths occur in India. Worldwide the major killers of children under five are pneumonia, diarrheal diseases (such as cholera), preterm birth complications, and birth asphyxia. Malnutrition and under nutrition are the underlying causes of one third of these deaths. In Sub-Saharan Africa malaria is responsible for sixteen percent of under-five deaths.[3]

Between 2011 and 2012 a famine in Somalia, caused by drought, high food prices and political conflict caused a large portion of an entire generation of Somali children to be lost. The United States Center for Disease Control and Prevention (CDC) estimates that 29,000 Somali children under the age of five had died within a ninety day time period.[4] En route to Mogadishu, thousands of families looking to escape the famine and find aid in the capital, lost child after child to starvation. This dire situation was further exacerbated by the inability of nations offering aid to gain access to the region, due to interventions on the part of Al Shabab, a rebel militia, which ordered those fleeing the famine back to their farms in light of incoming rain.

While making the nearly three week trek on foot to refugee camps, many parents had to make the difficult decision to leave a dying child behind in order to save a sibling still showing promise of survival. Some parents, not wanting to waste what little water they were carrying, denied a drink to children about to perish. Mothers lamented that they had to abandon children who were barely breathing in order to save themselves and their other children. One mother hurriedly buried her three year old son under dried branches in order to tend to her remaining five children. Many such children have been buried in make shift graves by mothers and fathers with barely enough energy to do anything more. The memory of these children, buried in shallow graves along the side of the road or wrapped in white clothes buried in refugee camps, will forever haunt their parents. Experts expect these parents to experience post-traumatic stress disorder, and interviews with these families reveal an overwhelming feeling of remorse.

The causes of high mortality in regions across the world and throughout history have been myriad; yet they fit a pattern. Factors that affect mortality rates include whether or not the child is breastfed and by whom, the education of the mother, the availability of clean drinking water, the ability to live in less densely populated areas, as well as socioeconomic status. Nevertheless, ignorance and neglect have been the chief causes of infant death up until the 1920s.

Historically, doctors were aware that infant deaths represented a large portion of the total mortality rate but did little to prevent it. Doctors were also aware that it was maternal ignorance that caused so many infant deaths; from offering improper food to neglect and unsanitary and unsafe living conditions. Physicians publicly stated that a practice as simple as avoiding cold baths for young babies could improve mortality. But mothers were being sent contradictory messages; on the one hand, infant death was common and to be expected, and on the other hand mothers were believed to be solely responsible for their children's health and well-being.[5]

Institutionalized Children

It has been noted that neglect or improper management caused half of the deaths of children who died in infancy.[6] However, there are specific conditions in a child's life which predict mortality. Institutionalized children (orphans, the abandoned, or foundlings), often died within a year of confinement. High mortality in "foundling homes" has not only been recorded in Medieval Europe but also in modern times. In present day China, due to the "One Child" policy, many infants (mostly girls or disabled boys) are abandoned on the road. While the statistics from China's census on these children are unreliable, some reports suggest that the mortality of children placed in Chinese orphanages were at least fifty percent in 1989.[7] Undercover reporting has exposed images and interviews describing the abuses and neglect of children left in these homes; children tied up, ill, and left to die alone. Of course, not all orphanages are so tragically administered. But it is the lack of individual care for young infants, among many other factors, which can facilitate an early death. Further, even when the conditions that prevail in these homes or orphanages are good, emotional and physical health is compromised, particularly for ill or disabled children. It is often children with special needs who are abandoned by parents that do not have the means to provide for them.

Abandonment and Illegitimacy

Many foundling hospitals opened in Europe during the Middle Ages to address the wave of infanticide. Thomas Coram fought for the creation of one such hospital in London after seeing exposed and dying infants in the street in the mid-1700s. In order to preserve the anonymity of the parents, a basket was suspended outside the hospital walls where unwanted infants could be placed. A bell was then rung to inform staff of new arrivals. London parents were so desperate to rid themselves of unwanted babies that a ballot system was devised in order prevent fights outside the gates. All abandoned children were admitted, which resulted in nearly 15,000 admissions, 10,000 of whom subsequently died. Eventually a decision was made to only admit children of single women. Ultimately, Britain passed *Offences against the Person* in 1861, which forbade abandonment of infants under two.[8]

It is generally well known that children born out of wedlock are vulnerable to higher rates of mortality. The research reflects the perspective that mortality is lower in societies that are accepting and supportive of unwed mothers and their children. In nineteenth century Scotland, for example, illegitimate children were not particularly vulnerable because of the absence of social stigma and the willingness of families to support single mothers. During economic hardship, however, infant mortality was eighty percent higher for illegitimate babies, likely due to lack of employment for unmarried women. Further, when mothers had to leave their babies with family to find work elsewhere, they had to wean their children early, putting them at higher risk of illness.[9]

Burial Clubs

The London General Bill of 1741 noted that fifty percent of all deaths were of children, thirty-three percent of whom were under the age of two. Causes of death included consumption, fever and tuberculosis. Around the same time, other cities in Europe experienced equally high mortality rates: in Barcelona sixty percent of deaths were children, Paris forty-five percent, Florence forty percent, and in Dublin a staggering eighty-eight percent.[10]

In these regions, mortality was so high that burial clubs were instituted. These clubs were equivalent to insurance for funerals; although, eventually it came to be discovered that some children were enrolled in more than one club. The death rates of these children were far higher than the rates of those not enrolled in any burial club (sixty-eight percent compared to thirty-six percent, respectively). To reduce the appeal of these burial clubs and any potential foul play, enrollment rules were changed to reduce the amount of the pay-out.

Breastfeeding and Wet Nurses

When a mother chooses to breastfeed her own child, she offers a level of protection against diseases to a very young infant unavailable through any other means. Breastfeeding had come in and out of vogue among the wealthy through different time periods, particularly in Europe. Yet poor mothers, if they had the ability to remain home with their infants (whether working for an income or not), generally nursed their children for as long as possible. A mother needing an income outside the home may have sent her infant out to a nurse, often to a region very different from the one in which the child was born in (e.g., from urban to rural). At least half of the infants sent out to a wet nurse died within a year. The causes of death were numerous, and the frequency with which these deaths occurred was suspiciously high. Deaths were often caused by the diseases wet nurses transmitted to their charges. A child being transferred from his birth home in an urban area to a wet nurse in the countryside would be exposed to diseases to which he had no immunity, even if his mother nursed him after birth. The wet nurse's milk would provide protections against diseases the child was exposed to while in her care, but once the infant returned home, his chances of benefiting from the antibodies in the breast milk were greatly reduced, as he was once again exposed to different diseases to which he and the wet nurse had no immunity.[11]

Wealthier women bringing nurses to their homes would experience similar problems. Many wet nurses were from poor areas, and living conditions were often unhealthy. Wet nurses brought diseases to children which they would not have been exposed to otherwise. Furthermore, nurses often breastfed multiple children and may not have had enough milk to adequately nourish them all. A nurse's poor diet would have further reduced her milk supply.[12]

In the nineteenth century, as wealthy women began to nurse their own children, poor women began to hire wet nurses so that they could work outside the home. As these services were very costly, a wave of abandonment and infanticide began. One infamous wet nurse, Margaret Elis Waters, took illegitimate babies into her home. When they died, as they so often did, she left them in the street. Mrs. Waters was subsequently executed for her crimes. This occurred in London in 1870, when over 244 babies were found in the streets. In another case, a Mrs. Martin was hanged for killing 500 newborns during her profession as a midwife. Many such midwives were convicted of killing newborns with opium cordials. These women were often jailed and ordered to wear two red stars -a sign of infanticide.[13]

Overlaying a child while breastfeeding or sleeping with an infant, was one of the most common causes of death for babies in the Victorian era. Fifty percent of children that died perished in this manner. This high mortality rate aroused suspicions of intentional smothering by both mothers and wet nurses.[14] Some historians have proposed that babies were sent to wet nurses expressly for the purpose of hastening their death.[15]

Despite the popularity of breastfeeding and nursing practices among both the rich and poor, there were many socioeconomic factors which may have mitigated their positive effects on mothers and babies. New mothers were often advised by midwives, popular among poor women, to avoid feeding colostrum to their babies (a pre-milk with antibodies present in the mother's breast right after birth) by not nursing their newborns for the first few days, contrary to the advice of physicians (who often serviced the wealthy during childbearing). Further, both the poor and wealthy tended to wean their children when the weather was fair. Disease was more rampant during the summer, and leaving children without the protective benefits of breast milk only contributed to high mortality rates, although in these instances the rich were more likely to survive than the poor.[16] For these reasons, it is difficult to make a linear connection between wealth and infant mortality—as circumstances and culture, beliefs of medical professional and other interfering factors would mitigate the effectiveness of breastfeeding.

Breastfeeding also has an effect on the length of birth intervals. A woman usually does not ovulate regularly, or at all, while breastfeeding. Therefore, there is an impact of previous infant mortality on current fertility. If an infant dies, thus halting breastfeeding, then the mother becomes fertile again immediately. An increase in fertility, however, can mean an increase in maternal mortality. While short birth intervals contributed to the poor health and inadequate care of a younger child, the presence of an older sibling had a positive effect on the mortality of a child under the age of one. Over the age of one, older siblings had a negative impact on mortality if the older siblings were brothers. Most importantly, though, a mother's death and her child's death were highly correlated.[17]

The professions of family members also had an impact on mortality if they affected whether a mother would not have to work outside the home, and would therefore be able to nurse and care for her own children. For example, in regions producing iron and steel, where only men could go to work, child mortality was low. In regions where textiles were produced or where there were dairies, mothers who could do this type of work left their children in the care of others. A working mother was highly correlated with child mortality; children always fared better if their own mothers nursed and cared for them.[18]

While breastfeeding was considered the norm among the working classes, in England for example, social class predicted mortality as socioeconomic status determined nutrition and access to medical facilities. Babies who were illegitimate or twins were likely to be weaned earlier; artificial feeding had a significant influence on the risk of death for those who died of diarrheal diseases. Accordingly, the appointment of a medical officer who supported breastfeeding, moderated illness caused by malnourishment, and educated mothers in proper infant feeding practices (such as avoiding giving children bad food or flour mixed with water in lieu of breast milk) was an essential predictive factor in lowering the childhood mortality rate.

Wealth and Mortality

As noted earlier, wealth is usually correlated with good health because of access to food and the ability to save money for crises. Additionally, the wealthy had better working conditions, medical support, social networks, and above all, knowledge. Nonetheless, in Britain from 1500 to 1950, child mortality was significantly higher among the elite and very wealthy than among commoners in London; albeit with some exceptions. Infant mortality was lower among laborers and paupers than other socioeconomic groups, even though the child mortality rate was higher. This unexpected dissimilarity may be explained by the fact that the wealthy often sent their children out to wet nurses. Wet nursing as has been discussed, was a determinant in infant mortality. Additionally, during outbreaks of disease, the wealthy would move away to equally unhealthy places. If a wealthy mother chose to nurse her own child and moved to another region she would not necessarily have the requisite antibodies present in her breast milk to help her infant to fight the diseases in the new region. Trade and travel also brought disease to the upper class.[19]

A similar phenomenon was observed in both nineteenth century Sweden and in Venice Italy, where the wealthy experienced high child mortality, while laborers realized lower child death rates.[20] Soren Edvinnson, a demographic researcher, explains that those who were laborers, or who were not land owners, could not afford milk; consequently mothers in these families had to breastfeed their children longer. Therefore, lower mortality rates occurred among laborers. Additionally, while not true of all poor families in nineteenth century Europe, in Venice the poor tended to live in open spaces –reducing the spread of infectious disease.

While the Catholic Venetians experienced relatively low mortality (twenty-five to thirty percent in the nineteenth century), infant mortality of Jewish children in the same region was even lower. Even the poorest Jews in Venice had lower mortality than the richest Catholics.[21] Lifestyle, in part, explains these differences; genetics, religious beliefs facilitating good health behaviors, personal hygiene, austere living, community welfare institutions and social cohesion, and prolonged breastfeeding (which also acted as birth control) all improved the mortality of Jewish, Venetian children. Other researchers have explained that the drastic differences in mortality between the two groups is due in part to Catholics demonstrating over mortality (twenty-five to thirty percent), that is, a higher mortality rate than expected, rather than Jewish under mortality, which was fourteen percent in the nineteenth century.[22]

Conflict

Not unexpectedly another major predictor of child mortality is warfare. In one example, during and after the Gulf War, from 1991 to 1998, 118–125 Iraqi children died per every 1000 live births. Mortality for children under the age of five was about sixty-three deaths per every 1,000 live births during time period preceding the Gulf War (1986–1990). The estimated number of excess deaths as a result of the Gulf War was between 400,000 and 500,000 (excess, meaning beyond what was projected in past population studies).[23]

In the thirteen years after the Cold War period, fifty-eight major conflicts were reported to have occurred in forty-six regions. Guha-Sapir and Gijsbert van Panhuis analyzed thirty-seven datasets on conflict related mortality. They found that while children in areas of conflict under the age of five were vulnerable, it is children over the age of five that have a higher risk of dying. These deaths are due to diarrheal diseases, malnutrition, respiratory illness and measles. In some regions such as Afghanistan, Somalia and the Sudan, the mortality rates were lower for children under the age of five during the period of conflict than it was before the conflict. It is possible that humanitarian aid, called in to respond to the conflict, improved access to food and health care for children that they would not have otherwise had. The type of war and international interest also impacts mortality.[24]

Parent Education Level

Parent education is often a significant predictor of socioeconomic status, and therefore, a predictor of high child survival rates. A mother's education significantly reduces the risk of infant mortality for the first child but not for others. A mother's education has the greatest effect when she has her first child because it improves her decision making and affects her ability to create a healthy environment for the entire family. A father's education reduces infant mortality for subsequent children, but not the first. This, in part, is due to the fact that education is a measure of the family's socioeconomic status; the lower the wealth, the higher the risk of mortality, particularly in the modern world.[25] Researchers also note that new interventions, such as better health care, tended to increase the inequality between mothers with higher education and those with none, but living in the same community, because the interventions initially would reach those who were already thriving.

The case of Afro-Brazilians is one example that demonstrates how racism can affect mortality, despite education. Although both Afro-Brazilians and whites have enjoyed significant improvements to living conditions, particularly with respect to health care, white children have experienced an unchanged 6.6 year advantage since the 1950s. (After Nigeria, Brazil has the largest African origin population of any nation; a result of the slave passage to North America.) Even though there are disparities between black and white mothers' education in Brazil, when controlling for this factor, mortality rates are still higher among blacks than whites.[26]

Other Causes of Mortality in Europe

Transitions such as birth, changes in feeding practices, and teething in the life of an infant are fragile periods. These events could leave the infant vulnerable to infection, especially if the child was weaned early from the breast. As noted previously, breastfeeding offered immunity from many fatal childhood illnesses, particularly respiratory diseases. Teething was generally cited as a cause of death because it coincided with weaning, but it was likely the subsequent offering of food not hygienically prepared, and the introduction of inappropriate foods, which may have caused diarrhea and ultimately death. Once a child reached nine months of age, it was more likely that human intervention could affect changes in mortality. Remarkably, an excess in infant male mortality was observed, even in regions where males are favored (that is, where females are more vulnerable to infanticide than males). During the first two weeks of life, males were almost fifty percent more likely to die than girls. The probability of male mortality rose again between the ages of three to eight months. Reasons cited for this disparity include the fact that boys tend to be less resistant to infection.[27]

Birth rank was another contributor to high infant mortality. Older mothers tend to give birth to weaker babies. Thus, the youngest child might be less likely to thrive than his older siblings (who had a younger mother). Accordingly, younger siblings were less likely to receive the benefit of a mother's energy and good health than older siblings. As noted previously though, the presence of an older sister available to help care for new babies could have a positive effect on mortality.[28]

Death clustering within families is another predictor of high mortality. When a child, particularly an infant, dies it leaves behind a "scarring effect" on the next child. Generally, clustering may be due to characteristics attributed to the mother, the family, or community such as genetics, access to clean water and health care. Scarring can also be attributed to a mother's grief and depression over the death of a child while pregnant with the next. Depression has been noted to cause physical symptoms such as insomnia and changes in appetite, which can affect the health of an unborn child. Further, when an infant's death hastens the weaning process, prematurely returning fertility and then pregnancy to the mother, her own health may be compromised because of nutritional depletion, again affecting the health of the new infant. The research has consistently stated that short birth intervals, less than six months, are detrimental to babies due to reduced maternal stores and competition with other children for resources and attention.[29] The optimal birth interval is eighteen months. Scarring is noted to be weaker in more developed regions, due to access to better facilities and resources, clean water and education.

Parent Education, Child Rearing, and Other Examples of Actions Taken to Improve Mortality

From 1890 to the early 1900s, in the United States, the child mortality rate for children under the age of five was twenty percent. Fifty-nine percent of those deaths were infant deaths. Primary causes of death were diseases such as cholera, diarrhea, pneumonia, meningitis and accidents. Thus, "germ theory" came to explain high mortality rates in many areas of the world. Additionally, impure milk and water were causes of death, although in communities where the mother worked at home and was able to breastfeed her children, illness was usually avoided or short-lived (as noted earlier in reference to European families).

In the 1800s smallpox killed one in three children in America. Inoculation to the disease, discovered by Edward Jenner in 1798, from cows with cowpox greatly alleviated the epidemic.[30] As parent education, access to vaccinations and public health policy improved, so did the mortality rate; however, a theme often heard about urban parents in the late nineteenth century was that they wailed for their child's death but were slow to take advice about their child's health.[31]

From 1760 to 1860 half of the children born in Russia did not survive to adulthood. While poor climate was blamed as a cause of death in Russia, other regions such as Norway, which has a harsher climate, had a lower mortality rate. Child-rearing practices such as cold (ice) water baptisms of newborns, swaddling, and improper feeding (e.g., foods in lieu of mother's milk) were ultimately deemed the cause of infant death. So devastating was the mortality rate, a Russian mother, who doted upon her infant, rocking it to sleep, was told "such exaggerated love…god will surely punish it".[32]

While ignorance about what children needed to survive in Imperial Russia may have been a major contributor to the high mortality rate, child murder (one of every eighty) was a shockingly common cause. It is possible that the actual murder rate was much higher since these crimes were only recorded if they were prosecuted in court. The government under Catherine the Great took action to reduce mortality rates. As in other regions of Europe, they created homes for orphaned and illegitimate children, released mothers and children from fasts prescribed by the Orthodox Church, and published manuals for child care.[33]

Changes in public health policy, coupled with parent education and sanitation innovations helped to enhance a child's ability to survive. In 1892 in France, several protective societies were established in order to help reduce mortality, albeit without much success. Pierre Budin, however, successfully opened a clinic for post natal care. Mortality was reduced from 178 to 46 per 1000 births in five years. In 1894 milk stations, *gouette de lait*, helped reduced mortality rates from diarrheal diseases from fifty-one to three percent.[34]

Public health policy also had caused acute changes in mortality in Aranjuez (near Madrid) Spain. For people born between the years 1871 and 1950, the life expectancy was approximately thirty years of age, and infant mortality was 200 per 1000 live births. In 1950, after the implementation of sanitation and health policies, life expectancy rose to above sixty-five years of age and mortality declined to eighty per 1000 live births.

There are limitations to interpreting historical medical documents by modern historians. Terminology often varies or is vague, and there may be a misunderstanding of the symptoms of diseases, which might cause a misdiagnosis.[35] Additionally, mortality rates and causes might be skewed due to the fact that seasonal diseases might be disguised by the uneven distribution of births (and deaths) throughout the year. For example, mortality during the eighteenth century in Europe peaked May through July, while it was low from December to February. The peak in late winter and early spring is associated with respiratory diseases due to the cold. A bad harvest could also affect a child's nutrition, which in turn could adversely affect his or her resistance to a disease. A peak in the summer was generally due to gastrointestinal disease caused by bacteria that thrived in food and water. Many contagious diseases, such as small pox, also peaked in the summer. Young infants who were fed artificially were even more susceptible to these diseases as they lacked their mother's immunity and were prone to exposure to contaminated foods, milk and water. Further, death as a result of respiratory disease was more likely to occur in the second six months of the first year of life. In a further demonstration of the "Matthew Effect" (the rich get richer, the poor get poorer), other researchers have shown that gastrointestinal disease, such as diarrhea, lowers the child's resistance to other infections. Again, breastfed children were less likely to submit to these types of diseases.[36] Living conditions also predicted mortality. Clean houses, open space between families (lack of overcrowding), access to clean water, and garbage collection systems were all aspects of communities for which child mortality was low.

From these data and anecdotes we can surmise a pattern of behaviors and environments that are conducive to the welfare of children, patterns that were used to inform public health policy and practice. As George Kent states in *The Politics of Children's Survival*, criticizing child survival programs, "good nutrition does not come from nutrition programs, and good health does not come from health services". Good health comes from a variety of elements: income, sanitary housing and food, as well as education, among as many other factors. Programs may help improve survival but it is the social structure and citizen's ability to command change that truly will improve health and therefore child mortality.[37]

2

Burial Pits and Ivory Beads

Prehistoric Children

In 2010 the earliest human remains ever discovered in the North American Artic were found in Upward Sun River. The cremated bones of a child, estimated to be about three years old, from 11,500 years ago (Late Pleistocene-Early Holocene Eras), were found in a burial pit within a semi-subterranean house. The child was discovered with his or her knees drawn up with arms to the side, indicating that the child was likely buried after death and not a victim of infanticide or cannibalism. Within the grave there was no evidence of burial ornaments; however, there were remnants of ochre which is often associated with prehistoric funeral rites. Remains of food items within the burial pit indicate that the pits' primary function was as a cooking hearth. After the cremation, the burial the pit was backfilled and apparently left undisturbed. The finding represents the "first evidence for behavior associated with the death of an individual" in northern North America.[1]

The historical literature on prehistoric children is limited, and records of deaths are dependent upon scientific reports produced by archaeologists and other scientists. Since we do not have the words of the prehistoric peoples to tell us how they felt about their children, we can deduce the meaning of burial practices not only based upon the accumulation of artifacts left behind, but on the features, spatial patterning and arrangement of the artifacts, as well as the social context (single graves, burial pits, or cemeteries) of the burial. Some of the most important cultural elements that allow us to understand prehistoric societies are their subsistence strategies, mobility (how often they move, how far, and in what social groupings), and their technology and tools (communal labor or specialists). These data also provide contexts for burials. The emotions of the parent, in relation to interpretation of archaeological excavations however, tends to be largely absent from the archaeological literature.[2]

Additional obstacles to interpreting childhood artifacts or the lack thereof, include the problem of how to identify what constitutes childhood in different time periods. Derevenski points out that childhood has diverse meanings in different cultures throughout history.[3] Often, in earlier societies the end of childhood may have been signified by the ability to live on one's own, while modern western young adults generally do not reach that milestone until far after developing physically into an adult. Additionally, skeletally mature children may not yet have the ability to reproduce, another marker of adulthood. For the purposes of this chapter, children are described as those under twelve years of age. This number generally defines the period of life before development into adulthood in much of the literature on children.

One example that allows us to see how subsistence strategies can be used to examine burial practices occurs in the Late Deccan Chalcolithic (~1000 BC) in what is now Maharashtra, India. Teresa Raczek argues that the evolution of daily food procurement practices, yet constancy of infant burial practices, is indicative of the social significance of mourning rituals. Performing traditional rituals in the face of crisis may have offered comfort to the grieving, particularly at a time of great social change. This can be seen in later pagan societies who had accepted Christianity yet returned to their traditional mourning practices in the face of death or illness.[4] Burial of the dead differs from other social practices in that it is not performed every day. Mourners might draw from commonly accepted funerary practices of their own culture, but will also personalize the burial or funeral for the individual. Therefore, funerary practices are reflective of both societal and individual values and conceptions of death and the deceased.[5]

The First Children

In 1924, the remains of the Taung Child, one of the first prehistoric children, were found in Bechuanaland (present day Botswana). The finding marked the discovery of a new species; the three year old child was determined to have originated from *Australopithecus africanus*, an African hominid that existed five to two million years ago. The child was found cast in limestone, thus very well preserved. He was likely killed by an eagle or another large predatory bird. In 1975 thirteen sets of remains were found in Hadar, Ethiopia. Four of them were of children under the age of five, and are believed to have evolved from the genus of the Taung child. This group has been referred to as the first family as "The presence of children in the group implies that *Australopithecus* functioned in communal and biological familial units".[6]

Between 200,000 to 400,000 years ago *Homo erectus* evolved into the new group *archaic Homo sapiens*. Skull bones thinned, the forehead became vertical, "brain volume increased and neurophysiological evolutionary qualities developed". With this development maturation delayed, and subsequently the need for maternal care increased. Through this increased nurturing the mother-child interaction emerged; a phenomenon characterizing *Homo sapiens*.[7] Evidence of this extended parenting is apparent in many of the child burial sites that have been discovered in the last century where infants and children are found ritually buried.

Burial Rituals

Ritual burial indicates not only societal beliefs, spiritual or religious, but also the amount of care attributed to a child during his or her lifetime, as well as the value placed on the child. Very often the grave goods buried with a child signify the expectation of what he would have been had he grown. Many of the following examples include the burial of tools associated with hunting in the graves of young male children. It appears that in typical burials children were found painted with either red or yellow ochre, as well as beads, pierced teeth and tools that may have implied "ascribed rather than achieved status" in Paleolithic societies.[8]

Several ritualized burials of prehistoric children have been found at Le Mousteir site in France. In one case, a young adult was found in the fetal position (a common position for the burial of Prehistoric peoples) with flints placed around his head, and with an ax and bones of cattle placed nearby. Nearby, the remains of a young child were found with a small flint placed over his heart. The presence of these tools might indicate expectations for these children to be hunters.[9]

Baby Amud, found in Israel in 1996, is the only example of an infant burial from Neanderthal society. The ten month old infant, ritually buried in a small niche of a cave nearly sixty thousand years ago, was found with the maxilla of a red deer on his hip. This particular burial illustrates the development of funeral practices among the Neanderthal species, as the offering of the deer's jaw is comparable to the burial of a two year old Neanderthal found with a piece of flint in Syria. Archaeologists do not know whether these funerals were the exception rather than the norm for child burials, however. Modern humans, who likely co-existed with Neanderthals at some point, share some common cultural characteristics with Neanderthals in that they symbolically and carefully buried their dead, including children.[10]

Mortuary study of Natufian infants and children has focused on whether the inclusion of grave goods, and decoration in particular, is indicative of social status, gender, or age. Researchers have argued that adults can garner a higher status by virtue of their abilities and personality, while children might inherit status through their family's wealth. As will be discussed further, children of many different societies were also often excluded from cemeteries, even when social status is clearly differentiated and also inherited. Some cultures, though, did not differentiate children from adults with respect to mortuary rituals. Among some groups of the European Mesolithic, infants were buried with the community. Additionally, the Ertebolle culture of southern Scandinavia buried newborns in communal graves along with grave goods, and at the Franchthi Cave in Greece, infants too were buried with the rest of their community.

In addition to burial with age and status-specific grave goods, it was not uncommon to find the dead covered in red ochre and wrapped in fur. Ochre had been frequently used to paint the bodies of the prehistoric dead. The use of red ochre on the dead is reflective of natural substances such as blood. Zagorska explains that "The presence of the color red in burials is regarded as being connected with the concept of death and with the preservation of the energy of life, providing magical force for the route to the world beyond."[11] Other uses of ochre observed among child and adult burials was the plastering of the face with blue or red clay mixed with red ochre, and amber colored rings found in the eye sockets. This particular ritual was used in burials found in Latvia and Finland. It appears that use of ochre ceased after the middle Neolithic period.[12]

Among some prehistoric peoples elaborate burials were common. An example of an extravagant burial was discovered at the site of Sungir in Vladimir, Moscow. The remains were excavated between the years 1957 and 1969, and represent the mid-upper Paleolithic period (about 24,000 years ago). The excavation, led by Otto Bader, revealed the graves of five individuals, two of whom were children. The male, approximately thirteen years old, and the female, seven to nine years old, were placed head to head with their hands crossed over their pelvises in what appeared to be a dwelling. A headless skeleton, which was presumed to be an adult male, was on top of the children. The male child was found with nearly five thousand ivory beads, which had been sewn into his clothes. Some sources estimate that it would take about an hour to make each ivory bead, indicating the high social status and wealth of the child's family. Additionally, his cap was inlaid with ox teeth, and a femur was found next him filled with red ochre. The female child was similarly adorned. In addition to their extravagant wardrobe, the children were found with lances and ivory discs. Another older adult male, buried within proximity and appearing to be of the same social group, was also decorated with ivory beads and teeth.[13]

While elaborate funeral rites were not uncommon in this time period, the double burial was unique in its extraordinary decoration of the children as well as their position in the grave. The burial position may have been constrained due to the inclusion of the grave goods, such as very long ivory spears, which would have inhibited a side-by-side position. Another more likely explanation, however, is supported by the discovery an ivory figure representing the same head-to-head position. This figure indicates, perhaps a sophisticated set of beliefs that is ensconced in mortuary behavior and tied to artistic representation.[14]

A more typical child burial from the same time period is represented by the Lagar Vehlo child discovered by Duarte and colleagues. The approximately four year old child, found on Iberia (Portugal), was heavily stained in red ochre and buried with two Littorino shells and four deer teeth. Archaeologists have determined that this child was related to the Neanderthal. This child represents the only well-recognized formal burial for a child from that period. The grave goods and burial treatment are similar to those found elsewhere in Europe.[15]

An analysis of children's bones found at the Gravettian triple burial site in present day Moravia, revealed that one of the children had a bone abnormality that may have been linked to a maternal diabetic condition. The burial of an "abnormal" child with a healthy one also indicates the existence of a complex set of beliefs related to funerary practices that supports acceptance of a diverse society, particularly when, among the ancient Romans for example, disabled children were generally victims of infanticide.[16]

While grave goods generally represented the gender and social status of a person, the evidence from different archaeological sites is contradictory. In the case of the Upper Paleolithic of the Central Russian Plain, Francis Harrold found no significant differences in grave goods (e.g., beads and tools) left with either adults or children in a sample of ninety-six burials. The graves of some adults and children contained many artifacts of wealth, while others did not, thus likely reflective of disparities in social status among individual societies or clans.[17] In the Early and Mid-Holocene Era of Northern Europe few children were buried with grave goods. Ten out of 100 child graves were found with bone tools for fishing and hunting.[18] Generally non-adults were buried with grave goods only if they were buried with an adult. In one example, in a Scandinavian cemetery at Vedbaek a mother and her newborn were found buried together with a pile of pendants made of red deer and wild pigs' teeth. The baby lay upon a swan's wing with a smaller wing placed on the baby's pelvis, indicating that it was a male.[19] In Mesolithic Zvejnieki (Latvia) non-adults appeared to be regarded in the same esteem as adults, as they were buried with tools.[20]

Burial Places

Monuments

The Cerny culture, in northern France, in the middle Neolithic (4300–4600 BC) built long barrows in which to bury the dead. These barrows varied in length, from twenty-five to 200 meters. Despite the amount of labor necessary to construct these monuments, and the degree of visual and cultural impact they had, generally only one person was buried in a barrow. It is assumed that these burials were indicative of a social organization structure, as other humans of this culture were buried in coffins or pits. Surprisingly, however, many older children were found buried in these monuments.

Most monumental burials in history seemed to be reserved for adults—usually reflecting an *acquired* status. Among the Cerny, the children found buried within the monuments are indicative of *inherited* status. While children under the age of one year were excluded from these burials, and young children were underrepresented, children between the ages of five and fourteen were overrepresented. Further, there were no significant differences between the quantity and quality of grave goods between the graves of adults and children. The grave goods included bones, flint arrow heads, and shells (found even with children younger than two who could not have possibly used these tools). Although Childe cautions against using grave goods to ascribe wealth, among the Cerny a hunter is of an exalted status—and the grave goods are those associated with hunters. As mentioned previously, subsistence strategies can reflect beliefs about burials, although the Cerny were an agricultural society. The inclusion of arrows in some of the child graves indicates a predetermined role for these children as hunters or predators. Further, were no differences in grave goods of children buried in the monuments and in the flat graves (pits and coffins). Researchers have been unable to explain the differences between the children buried in these two places.[21]

Cillini

Nyree Finlay argues that infants were treated differently during the Neolithic and Early Bronze age with respect to the location of their burials. The choice of burial location for infants appears to mirror the treatment of other persons in other eras that were excluded from usual mortuary practices, such as those who had committed suicide, victims of famine, or non-Christians. As will be discussed in Chapter 4, Ireland has a long history of burying unbaptized children separately from those buried within the church yard. These separate burial spaces were called *cillini* or *Killeen*, derived from Latin for little church—*cella.* Finlay cautions against attributing adults in the category of other (suicide, non-Christian, etc.) just because they are buried within the *cillini,* as many sites may have two burial contexts together from different eras in history (e.g., one from the prehistoric era and one from the Middle Ages).[22]

Meanings of infant burial in prehistoric Ireland, namely during the Neolithic and Bronze Ages, is in part dependent upon interpretation of placement of remains. The site of Fourknocks in Meath County is a late Neolithic passage tomb with three chambers. Both Fournocks and Fournocks II have been analyzed with respect to differential treatment of children and adults. Children were often buried on the periphery, while adults, who were cremated, were laid to rest in the center.[23] A predominant characteristic of infant burials "reflects reuse or at least chronologically later phase of activity than most of the adult cremations." At one of the sites cremation deposits have fragments of inhumations within the chambers and passage. It is possible that these distinctive passage burials are symbolic, as the placement is symbolic, "the passage itself is a threshold between the domain of the living and the ancestral dead."[24] The evidence surrounding the infant burials, for example remnants of animal bones and cremation, suggest that the infants were removed and reburied as a symbolic gesture.

Uncharacteristic of young children found at this site, an older child was found in a crouched position (a common burial position) with a grave good – a food vessel. Yet another child was found to be buried so that he or she disturbed the burial of a younger child. This provides further evidence of differential treatment for older children, as young children were generally only found to be buried within the passageways. While myriad reasons exist for separate burials of infants and young children, some archaeologists insist that the characteristics of these sites point to infanticide, in part because many of the sites described above were already in the process of destruction or decay at the time of the burials.[25] Mother and infant burials, on the other hand, appear to have been treated more delicately. In one case a presumed mother is buried near a fetus with a boar's tusk. In keeping with tradition, she was cremated and her infant inhumed with her.[26]

Burials in Homes

Death played a large role in the domestic lives of early Neolithic people. They often buried their dead under house floors, and represented death in the décor of their homes. In many other regions of the prehistoric world infants were often buried beneath house floors. In Vlasac and Lepenski Vir (southeastern Europe), during the Mesolithic and early Neolithic eras, adults could be found buried with neonates. The bones of the fetuses or newborns would be covered in red ochre over the groin area, or with Cyprinidae teeth placed in the groin area, signifying concern for the family, and the mother in particular. An older infant buried with fifty perforated snails may reflect "its stage of social embodiment" differing greatly from that of newborns.[27] Often young infants were buried with the head toward the southeast, parallel to the Danube, the head pointing downstream. Some infants were positioned in such a way to indicate that they had been placed in a bag before being interred in burial pits. While burial within homes was common, neonates, who had previously been buried with adults around open air hearths, were later buried under a red limestone floor in the rear of the building, suggesting a major social and ideological restriction in the region. Burial of a child within the house allows the spirit to protect living and future children, and it is also intended to induce fertility. In keeping with this practice, the Saracatsans of the Balkans would place a newborn or a miscarried fetus in a bag of salt and hang it above its parents' bed for forty days until it dried out, where it was then buried in a corner of the hut.[28]

The people of the early Neolithic *Linienbanderkeramik* (LBK) culture lived on sites, which became mounds, where the LBK lived repeatedly. Children were not often buried in cemeteries in this culture. Rather their remains were found most often inside the settlements—indicating a close tie between the living and the dead. Interestingly, infants were not found in the settlement or in the cemeteries. Because of the high number of women and children buried in the homes, some scholars conclude that persons who were of insufficient status were relegated to house burials.[29] Another explanation for house burials of women and children are that these two groups are often associated with domesticity. Further, within and without the home, food is often a symbol for the relationship between mother, or caregiver, and child. Scott cautions readers from identifying practices which are different for males and females as being important and unimportant, respectively.[30]

At the Neolithic site of Catalhoyuk's (modern day Turkey) foundation and threshold burials have also been found in dwellings. In ancient societies foundation sacrifices were made to assure the stability of a building, and often included sacrifices of living children. In prehistory, however, these discoveries do not indicate sacrifice or infanticide as they were typical burials.[31] Further, burials within homes were usually through a limestone floor, which would cause damage. Therefore, this practice did not provide evidence of foundation sacrifices, which would have occurred before the house, and the floor in particular, was complete.

Several types of special burials have been identified for prehistoric children in Catalhoyuk. These burials are different from those that had been typically placed beneath a floor on the north side of the house (although neonates were found on the south side in a basket near the hearth; indicating the spiritual significance of the direction). Foundation burials, with neonates or stillborn children buried with shell and obsidian, stained with red ochre, and shrouded in a basket set high in the wall are among one special type. Small handprints found painted in red over a bull's snout on a wall suggests the religious symbolism of infants in the room. Foundation burials were often tied to the "cost of the community as sacrifice". Threshold burials represented change of space use and ritual burial. They were often found out in the open, as in a courtyard. This placement is significant visually as it allowed for public access. As noted earlier foundation burials in prehistory do not necessarily signify infanticide; however, in some cases infants and young children found at the threshold, at the point of construction of the building, seem to point to an unnatural death.[32] A threshold burial signifies liminal status. Therefore a sacrifice made in this space is meant to purify and consecrate a doorway, since crossing a threshold was considered dangerous to one's health. Children represented a purity and closeness to the supernatural world. While it is unclear whether they were buried postmortem or as a result of infanticide, the sacrifice was meant to fortify the home for siblings.[33]

Jar Burials

During the Pottery Neolithic and Chalcolithic jar burials were prevalent. Infant burials were rather elaborate considering that is was a time known for few onsite burials. Jar burials are interpreted as a simulation of a womb. Most jars were laid on their sides but some were inverted, with the neck opening downward—perhaps simulating a rebirth. Jars found on and below floors, corners, thresholds or by wells, generally included children from fetus stage to ten years old. Jars with long necks and narrow openings were reserved for older children. Neonates had wider mouth vessels, indicating a "sentimental" burial.

As noted previously, among prehistoric groups it was often difficult to ascertain whether a burial was the result of a ritual sacrifice. In Southern Levant, many of the excavated remains were identified as males. Different interpretations of the burials could reveal ritual sacrifice of males in general or firstborn males; or they could signify sentimental burial of beloved children combined with the particular locations of the children.[34] African jar burials hint at sacrifice, given the location of the deposit and the lack of grave goods; this in addition to evidence of violence, dismemberment in particular. During this same period, jar burials were prevalent in the Near East. Burial location combined with the use of the vessels appears to indicate a call for rainfall and prevention of drought. Orrelle also suggests that this culture was involved in "elite" beverage production, as evidenced by the diverse use of drinking vessels for many purposes. The practices of the people of the Pottery Neolithic in Southern Levant share some common attributes to those in Neolithic Northern Sudan in that a fetus may be found in a pot in relation to the house enclosure, and a stillborn baby, who had not yet "drawn a breath", were buried just outside the outer wall. In Zimbabwe, premature or aborted babies were buried in a jar and placed in the sand of a dry river bed. When it rained, the sand and the baby were washed out from the jar like a birth so that, symbolically, the mother could get pregnant again after the baby was "delivered".[35]

In the Chalcolithic period in Northern Levant a necropolis of jars and other burials was unearthed. Nearly forty percent of the burials were children, and included grave goods of metal hooks, cups, weapons, bone and ivory items, and art objects. Non-typical jars contained infants, buried vertically, and ten percent of these jar burials were found near or under houses.[36] Some pots were used specifically for burial, while others were reused cooking vessels. Cooking and eating often took place in the same place as burial, as exemplified by the finding described in the opening of this chapter. Babies' vessels were circular while older children were in jars; as discussed earlier the different shapes were symbolic.

In addition to jar burials, children could also be found inhumed. Occasionally cemeteries with single burials could be found in the Mediterranean or Near East, but these were less common. When multiple burials occurred, it was usually with several other children, or with a woman assumed to be the mother. Infants at times could be found in baskets with distinctive grasses indicating that the receptacles were not used for household chores; therefore, ascribing these items as common burial vehicles for the very young. It is important to note that interpretation of some burial practices is confounded by newer burials on top of older ones.[37]

Status of Children in Burials

Among the various excavation sites that have revealed the discovery of prehistoric children and adults, there are many clues as to the mortality as well as the social status of children. For example, age related mortuary practices have been documented at many archaeological sites among different cultures; there might be a special area for young children or grandparents. The lack of mortuary behavior is also telling. In late pre-pottery Neolithic no specific funeral treatments were applied to neonates who were either stillborn, or were born and died shortly after birth. A large number of infant burials were found at the Khirokitia site. Le Mort argues that this anomaly may be explained by several possibilities. First, this society may have practiced mortuary behaviors that allowed for better preservation of infant skeletons than of other societies. It is also possible that infanticide was practiced; however, in order for this hypothesis to be proved, sex ratio must be established to determine whether the sample of infants represents a typical population (and therefore not indicative of infanticide). Finally, this large sample might reflect an epidemic affecting the very young at the time.[38]

Among some populations no differences may be found in the treatment of children. Of hunter-fisher-gatherers of the Dnieper Rapids of Ukraine, children "could be integrated into social structure from an early age" as evidenced in the archaeological study of burials of sub adults in the region.[39] Children played an active role in "subsistence tasks" and were recognized as having an elevated social status, for which burials identical to those of adults were warranted. Similarly, child burials were rare in the Greek Neolithic period. Child mortuary practices were similar to those of adults until the late Neolithic, therefore it is impossible to interpret children's status in Greek Neolithic Society.[40]

Child burials became more visible in the Bronze Age, although evidence of very few infants and young children can be found. At Mokrin, for example, not one infant under the age of one was found in the cemetery, and the only intact infant burial of this group was found under a house floor.[41] In East Manych, too, during the Bronze Age, few infants and young children were found. Children may have been poorly preserved and infants not buried until they reached the social status associated with weaning or walking. Those who were buried were found with an older adult called a "child's guide" either in the same burial structure or barrow. Some of the burials may indicate unnatural deaths as the bones of the adults were disarticulated—indicating that burials had been disturbed and re-deposited in a collective burial, or that the bodies were dismembered purposefully. A prestigious burial on the other hand might incorporate a deposit of the remains of a newborn as there were a high percentage of children under the age of two buried with an adult. Positioning of the children against the adults was always practiced. There were no instances of an adult and child of the same gender buried together, nor were there triple burials or individuals belonging to the same age group. These data indicate that there was a relationship between marriage and burial rites, as pre-adults (adolescents) had no "child's guide".[42]

Infanticide among Prehistoric Groups

Fire brought about the institution of cooking to the *Homo erectus* which facilitated the development of the parent-child relationship. For example, cooked food became a consistency that young children could eat in lieu of breast milk, thus hastening weaning and minimizing birth spacing. It introduced the division of labor as women cooked the food, and reinforced pair-bonding and the creation of the family unit. Further, the bond between mother and newborn that formed created a sense of empathy within the mother. Babies "elicited nurturing", not only from their own mothers but from other maternal figures within the community. Infant sharing among communities of women also facilitated what Hrdy postulates as "a need to help". The evolution of family and maternal love aside, infanticide was widely practiced when the demands of mothering exceeded the abilities of the mother. Infanticide was intra-familial. Thus, this collaborative parenting seemed to support infanticide as parents' personal responsibility and concern for their children was diluted by the responsibility and concern by the community.[43]

Infanticide, by reasons of physical defect or lack of maternal resources evolved into infant sacrifice by way of Paleolithic magic systems. Dervin postulates that as the cooking hearth became the center of the community, it evolved into the altar. Early humans began to communicate with spirits that they began to believe could be appeased with sacrifice in order to avoid natural disasters. Consequently, evidence of cannibalism was also observed.[44]

Parental grief, if one wants to ponder whether it existed among prehistoric peoples, could be a complicated matter. Neanderthal families were not nuclear in the sense of the word as we know it today. As noted above, in prehistoric societies parenting of a child was often shared by the community. There was cross-mothering, cross-siblings (cousins), and men often swapped women.[45] Mothers may have had several partners who could have been the potential fathers of her children. In fact, it was in her best interest to lay with more than one male while pregnant. Some anthropologists contend that when two males have lain with a woman just before or at pregnancy, those men would consider themselves co-fathers, which is also termed "partible paternity". An additional father can help a baby survive. On the other hand, a male who invests time and energy to feed a helpless infant must be sure of its paternity, or the genes of another male may benefit. While infanticide was very common, the "loss of a wanted child is enormously costly to any human mother, making it best not to divulge but precisely to confuse accurate paternity information..."[46] Thus making the case for a mother to take several partners during pregnancy, particularly if one of them proved to be a poor father or dies.

The population explosion of *Homo sapiens* is inconsistent with female tolerance of infanticide. Large numbers of large-brained, slow to develop children required quality child care in order to be raised to maturity. Thus the bonds that were cultivated between parent and child explain, for the most part, the move away from a culture of infanticide.

The exclusion of babies from newborn to one year of age at many sites has concerned archaeologists and anthropologists, even as various explanations have given way to assumptions of cultural practices. The absence of many infants from the archaeological record has been explained with the possibility that the remains of infants and children are more susceptible to disintegration after burial. However, the Belleview study found that the skeletons of infants and children do not decay more rapidly than those of adults.[47] Sub-adults, however, may be buried in more shallow graves, and therefore more likely to be disturbed or destroyed.

Given the evidence, it appears that in many cultures, infants were not always ascribed a status commensurate with that of older children and adults. Therefore, they were buried elsewhere. Scott warns that interpretations of burial sites which lack infants, or sites where urn burials are common should not simply be explained as evidence of infanticide. Cultural contexts must be considered, and caution should be exercised before observing patterns where they do not exist. Children and infants in particular are often given a liminal status which precludes them from adult and adolescent funeral rites and burial locations.[48]

3

Burials at Night

Children from Ancient Civilizations

Archaeological evidence excavated from what is known as Mesopotamia, between the Tigris and Euphrates rivers, suggests that the Sumerians and Akkadians, the first civilized people, cared for their children; although evidence also suggests that first born children were often sacrificed. Further, the Sumerian code of laws, *ana ittisu,* which stated laws such as the fact that parents could give up children when it suited them, makes it difficult to interpret the ancient society's concern for children. These contradictory ideals, which apply to many of the societies discussed here, illustrate the extent to which parental love is both dynamic and complex in the ancient world.

Evidence of Parental Concern

It is clear from the artifacts and writings left behind that Egyptian children were warmly cared for. Young children from all social classes were treated equally until school age. The tombs of children were often found with mummified pets to go with them on their journey to the afterlife. Premature infants, as well as their umbilicus, were also mummified. This practice leads historians to believe that Egyptian parents hoped that their infants would go on to be nourished through the umbilical cord, grow, and live the life they were meant to live. The Egyptians called the soul of a child *ba,* a bird with a human head.[1]

In ancient Egypt abandonment and infanticide were rare. In fact, the Egyptians were well known for rescuing abandoned infants. The Egyptian code of law implicitly made provisions for the protection of the unborn. For example, parents were required to include abandoned infants as heirs to an estate.[2] Additionally, murder of children was punished in such a way as to incite the community. When a murder of a child occurred, particularly if the parents were the offenders, the murderer was required to "embrace the murdered children in [his or her] arms for three days and three nights".[3] Other ancient civilizations punished child murder similarly. For example, the Hittites in Anatolia (modern day Turkey) required a man to replace any child that he had killed, while the Franks fined those who committed infanticide. The penalties varied depending on the age and gender of the child. Unnamed newborns, for example, commanded less of a fine than a child older than ten years of age or a pregnant girl.[4]

Among Minoan-Mycenaean families, children of commoners were buried in caves or within the home, perhaps because parents hoped that the children would be reincarnated again into the same family. Alternately, noble children, like their parents were buried within tombs and often dressed in elaborate gold costumes.[5] While these practices indicate that Minoan-Mycenaean parents commemorated the deaths of their children, as with many other ancient societies, they also legalized abandonment. For instance, if a woman was separated from her husband and he did not accept the infant as his own, legally she could expose the child.

The Etruscans, generally described as an immoral, scandalous society, commonly left behind depictions of loving, familial relationships in burial monuments. Children, and adults, were cremated and placed in house-like tombs with all of the accoutrement of a comfortable home (clothing, lighting, food, etc.). Pictures of Etruscan children could also be found carved into a mother's sarcophagi.[6]

Among the ancient Karelians (of Finland), people believed that the soul flew from the body in the form of a bird or butterfly. To prevent the deceased from returning home, the family of those buried within a cemetery would place a lopped off tree as a barrier to the home. It is believed that huge tombstones served the same function: to stop the dead from haunting survivors (who may have felt guilty because of their survival). Alternately, burial in the home suggests that the spirit was being summoned back into the body. Like many other ancient cultures, the Karelians buried their dead with items they might need on their journey, such as tools. Other burial practices included painting girls' coffins red and boys' coffins blue.[7]

In ancient Japan evidence exists of the child as a symbolic focus in mortuary practice. Mizoguchi demonstrates this phenomenon using two cemetery sites during Fukuoka Prefecture in the Northern Kyushu region of Japan: Nagaoka and Kuriyama during the Yayoi period (3rd to 1st century BC). In Nagaoka cemetery younger children were buried in jars and often placed inside adult pits or pits for older children, which reflected structure within the society. Over fifty percent of those buried in this manner were infants. Multiple children interred with one adult indicated that a family died together. Or perhaps, as practiced in other cultures when the care giver of the children died, infanticide was committed. Another explanation for these multi-generational interments is that the children were buried with ancestors so that they may be cared for in the afterlife. Interestingly, the visual arrangement of the burial grounds was constructed to facilitate the perception by mourners of a sense of community as the view of graves was widened as the funeral procession approached. At Kuriyama children were treated as adults, and entombed in jar burials. Clusters of burials indicated familial grave sites and a focus on the household unit. Kuriyama, contrary to the cemetery structure of Nagaoka, was arranged so that the mourner's gaze would be drawn to the last grave. Children selected to be buried in this cemetery were thought to be successors to a group leadership.[8]

Romans

In Common Era Roman Italy only babies less than forty days old were permitted to be buried within the town walls, as they were not considered to be developed enough to cause "religious pollution". The Ancient Romans had special customs for children who died either before the appearance of teeth or before their fortieth day of life. They were always buried (never cremated on a funeral pyre) in a Suggrundarium, a grave under the family home.[9] Infants were far less often memorialized than older children, and certainly not at a level comparable to the mortality rate. Although, when honored, Roman children were commemorated in an elaborate style for which there was no parallel, in earlier or later societies, before the twentieth century.[10]

The ancient Romans were superstitious and feared the dead, which was reflected in the way they buried those who had died a bad death, much like in other ancient societies. The very young and those born prematurely were buried at night in a family ceremony. Children had no social identity and a marginal status, thus the burial could not be a social event.[11] Children were, however, carefully buried, neatly laid out, and wrapped in shrouds or placed in a coffin. When they were cremated, the remains were placed in urns. Graves were held down with large stones or pot lids to prevent a child from "ghostly walking". The graves were unusually secure so that the child would pass safely to the afterlife and not escape to haunt the living. In one example, a baby wrapped in a colored shawl with aromatic resin around his face was found with a box of pipe clay figures on top of the coffin in order to hold down the lid.[12]

The ancients had a long history of inscriptions on tombs or stelae (similar to a tombstone). The inscription generally indicated the site of the tomb, where siblings were to be buried, as well as the names and titles of the dead. Later the inscriptions began to include a prayer and biography of the deceased. Inscriptions on tombs for children often included expressions such as *dulcima et amantissi* (expressions of futility, and pride). They might also include childhood sculptures illustrating the parent's love for the child. In one example, the epitaph of a twelve year old Arcadian girl indicates that her parents wished she had died younger; before they had grown so attached to her.[13] Vikings, too, left runic stele (tombstones) which often did not provide any more information than the first name of the deceased. One rune stone stated: "There will not be a greater memorial, mother made after her only son."[14]

While wanted children may have been carefully buried, in ancient Rome a family was only permitted to have three children. This number included at least one female. Ultimately, fathers made the decision as to whether or not children should be kept after birth. In one often quoted example, a letter from a husband to his expectant wife about the impending birth of their child says "if it is a girl expose it".[15] Although, according to the law, all children must have been permitted to live until at least three years of age, ill or abnormal infants could be exposed after five witnesses confirmed and approved the child's condition. Violation of these laws was punished by a fine equal to half of a family's estate. Despite laws against infanticide, the practice was often a topic of humor in comedies such as the *Girl from Samos*.[16]

Among the Romans, the infant mortality rate was about thirty-three percent, and one third of children were dead by age ten. This percentage excludes children who were abandoned.[17] Malformed infants, when born, were not treated. Instead they were neglected and left to die when perhaps, with some care, they would have lived. Disabled or malformed children were considered a sign of gods frustrated by the failings of humans. They were drowned after birth, or killed by fire when the anomalies were obvious. It was thought that the regular practice of killing abnormal children removed a defective gene from the evolutionary process;

less obvious abnormalities, however, went undetected and continued to course through bloodlines.[18]

The discovery of the remains in twenty different sites, from the fourth century BC to the first century AD, in classical Rome indicates a change in view of the afterlife by the Dacians, those who lived there before the Romans. From five to three BC two thousand graves were found, while later, from two BC to one AD, only 150 were found. Most remains were discovered in cemeteries or a settlement, and the rest in field of pits, in isolated pits, or in homes. Fragments of skeletons or isolated bones have been found in sacred areas indicating ritual burials. Many of these burials were comprised of children ages newborn to seven, although some field pits contained children of mixed ages, signifying family burials. Because no grave goods were found, although older children might have had some clothing or jewelry, the site was indicative of a children's necropolis. Other burials, however, pointed to unnatural deaths. From two BC to one AD, children were found buried in one pit, in unusual positions, showing evidence of violence. In another example, a child was buried in the proximity of a man and a young girl, placed deliberately in a sexual position, which suggested sacrifice.[19] In another transition of child burial practices, from the second to the third century AD, all children in a settlement were buried, but most adults were cremated. The simplest explanation for this change over the course of six to eight centuries is that when Roman rule commenced in the area, there was less sacrifice of children and more burials — perhaps to religious beliefs.[20]

While there may have been less sacrifice when Roman rule began, some findings point to infanticide on a large scale. For example, at a Roman villa in Hambleden, in Buckinghamshire, Britain, ninety-seven young infants, mostly full-term newborns, were found buried close together under walls or courtyards. Many were buried in a cloth, wrapped in a bundle. The graves were unmarked, so on occasion one infant might be found on top of another. Alfred Heneage Cocks, who excavated the site in 1912, proposed that these burials took place at night in secret, and that they were, therefore, likely evidence of illegitimate births. Archaeologists postulate that the site is perhaps an ancient brothel, and babies were killed and buried directly after death in order to keep the mothers working. Scott, however, argues that this conclusion is based on the social context of post-medieval England, in which women killed their bastard newborns, and not that of Roman Britain.[21] Further, unmarked graves of children are sometimes interpreted as a parent's lack of concern. But even in ancient societies funerals were costly, and the services of wailing women or an undertaker needed to be paid for. During a time when it was common to lose several children, the cost of a funeral for a child may have been too much for some families. In present times, in some communities parents who seek out local associations to help pay for a burial must leave the grave unmarked by a headstone. For this reason, Scott argues that it might be more useful for us to look at family groups to determine infant and child status in burials.

Ancient Athens

In ancient Greece children were rarely commemorated at their death. When parents were permitted to bury their children, it was within the house. Kurtz and Boardman contend that based upon this evidence parents lacked concern and did not demonstrate grief for their children when dead.[22] On the other hand, Binford, an archaeologist, argues that burial of children within the house may be interpreted as a form of "sympathetic magic, a statement that the household welcomes children; or a mark of the parents unwillingness to give up a child completely".[23] As among the prehistoric and indigenous peoples (see Chapters 2 and 7, respectively), as well as the ancient Romans, burial within the house was symbolic; the child's spirit both induced fertility and protected siblings. As discussed further in Chapter 10, in response to grieving parents in ancient Greece, academics and public figures often advised parents to moderate their anguish. Cicero is quoted as saying "If a child dies young, one should console himself easily".[24]

Studying 2,000 child burials from 1100 to 0 BC in Ancient Athens, Houby-Nielson notes that infants and children were carefully buried in cemeteries designated and devoted to the young, often in view of the Sacred Road.[25] Additionally, great care was exercised in preparing the burial of the child. Women cared for the corpses, and were also mourners and trained lamenters. There were differentiations between the burials of an infant, a young child, and an older child (up to age nine). Infants were buried in jars, closed with a stone or covered with a slab. Food was left with the child so that he or she would be nourished in the afterlife. The young child was buried in household terra cotta basins, or in wood coffins or pits. The older child was buried in a cist tomb. To put these burial practices within the perspective of cultural practices of the time, it is important to note that most adults were cremated up until the sixth century. In addition to being buried with nourishment, toys and gender specific grave goods (e.g., swords, makeup, and needles) accompanied young children. Tiny utensils and jugs for drinking were also left with infants and children. Older children were often buried with jewelry. Over the fifth century the burials of infants and young children increased greatly. Newborns in particular were entombed under fireplace stones. Often this practice indicated the desire by parents to care for the infant's grave or to have the soul of the child reincarnated into the next baby born to the family.[26]

Among the Huns at the beginning of the fourth century BC, when Athens was no longer independent, traditional infant and child cemeteries disappeared. The reduction of burial rites for young children was related to the decline of political ideology and the increased appearance of relief decorated grave stones, often commemorating children who were not given a formal burial.

Anglo Saxons

For the early Anglo-Saxons, between the fifth and seventh centuries, invaluable primary source data is drawn from excavated cemeteries; in particular Audrey Meany's catalog of 25,000 graves. This source not only provides evidence of burial rituals, but also highlights what is lacking. Pagan Anglo Saxons had two main forms of burial rituals: cremation (ashes often placed in burial pots) and graves (inhumation). But there appears to be a dearth of children in Anglo-Saxon graves.[27] One reason for this absence is because of the common practice of cremating Anglo Saxon children. Additionally, cremation sites often contained the ashes of more than one person. There was also an uneven distribution of burials across ages. Infants, for example, barely left any trace in the archaeological record which may due to burial practices that inhibited preservation of remains. Other than infanticide and improper disposal of remains, infants and young children might have been buried in shallow graves which may have made them susceptible to being dug up in excavations, or they may have been buried in separate cemeteries.

Of those graves identified, most lacked decoration. While grave goods often included jewelry, accessories of clothing, and weapons, no type of burial or grave good is associated with Anglo Saxon children, a practice differentiating this group from other ancient societies. Crawford offers some explanations for this anomaly. First, it is important to note that artifacts buried with the dead were often age related. While the pattern of child burial may not be visible to modern societies, is it not visible because we do not understand it.[28] During this period, a ten year old child was considered mature; therefore, these adolescents were buried with adult rituals and grave goods, but identified as non-adult by archaeologists. Further, it is possible that if toys were buried with children, they would not survive as they were often created from ephemeral materials such as cloth and flowers.

In keeping with the perspective of adolescents as adults, at an excavated site in Kent, some children were buried with child sized artifacts usually reserved adults, such as brooches and spear heads, while young girls might have been buried with jewelry and gold; perhaps their bridal gifts. One infant was buried with a 'mammiformed pot with a teat' (a pot in the form of breast, an ancient baby bottle of sorts) which likely indicated a child who was unable to nurse. A woman presumed to be his mother, was found buried nearby, a boar's tooth buried between them (which indicates a relationship between the sets of remains).[29]

Sacrifice and Infanticide in the Ancient World

Not all ancient civilization revered children, living or dead. The Phoenicians exhibited the most notorious example of child sacrifice. In Carthage between the years 800 BC to 146 BC, when the Romans destroyed the city-state now known as Tunisia, large numbers of children were sacrificed by fire in order to ensure military and financial success. Often parents chose their best-loved child, many times infants only a few weeks old, to be sacrificed in order to appease the god Baal so that they would be the recipients of good fortune; a successful shipment of goods for example. Children were placed in the arms of a bronze statue where they then fell into a brazier. Music was performed in order to drown out the sounds of crying mothers. In the kingdom of Sheba infants were sacrificed and cannibalized as well. Sacrifices of both children and adults were made to the planet gods. An example of the cruelty that occurred included an infant who was "boiled and deboned…rolled in flour, oil, saffron, raisins, and spices and then oven-baked…[then] eaten by the priests during the ceremony to Shemal."[30] In many of these societies infanticide and human sacrifice were practiced in preparation for war. The burial grounds where these infants were laid to rest were called tophets, and can be found in other regions of the world such as Marsala, Sicily.[31]

Additionally, Plutarch reported that the Carthaginians, presumably the wealthy or those who had no children, purchased babies from the poor and cut their throats. A mother could not or did not cry out lest she lose the fee she was paid for relinquishing her child for sacrifice.[32] In ancient Rome parents were paid to keep children alive (that is, to not commit infanticide), the Christians, accused by the Romans of dealing in child sacrifice, noted the hypocrisy: "How many, do you suppose, of those here present who stand panting for the blood of Christians -how many, even, of you magistrates who are so righteous against us-want me to touch their consciences for putting their own offspring to death".[33]

As noted previously, the ancients were fearful and superstitious when it came to burial of the dead. For example, some societies practiced foundation sacrifice, where the remains of a dead child were buried within the foundation of a new building as a means of (spiritual) fortification. While it is believed that these types of sacrifices often only included the remains of miscarried or premature infants, Egyptians were also reported to have buried children alive when a parent or care-giver passed away so that the parent could care for the child in the afterlife.[34]

In ancient Greece and Rome there were no laws against abandonment until the fourth century. Some ancient scholars believed that men should be able to do whatever they wanted with their children, others, like Seneca and Aristotle expressed that infanticide should be reserved for the deformed or sick. Infanticide and abortion were used as birth control, the former being the preference, as the latter could put the mother at risk and often failed. Infanticide of this nature was not considered a crime, since a child did not "exist" until his father accepted him.[35] Despite what appears to be general acceptance of exposure and infanticide, several writings from the ancient have been found which speak against these practices. Musonius Rufus, who wrote *Should Every Child That is Born be Raised?*, stated that brothers are useful and should be spared. Justin Martyr, like many religious figures, lamented against exposure and infanticide and expressed that children should be seen as gifts from god. Finally, among the Trojans, Hadrian appointed a superintendent of child welfare in order to revoke the long held right of father's to expose children he did not want. As a result of Hadrian's appointment the sale of children and castration was also prohibited.[36]

In Ancient India infanticide was practiced due to the difficulty of marrying daughters to good families, among other reasons. If a family did not want a female child, after the infant was delivered the mother might put opium on her nipple, which the infant would inhale while nursing, causing it to die.

While infanticide was very common in early China (discussed further in Chapter 11), particularly during the Han dynasty (206 BC to 220 AD), certain death rites were attributed to children and infants. It was commonly believed that the dead came back to "haunt" the living. For example, evidence from an excavation at Shuihudi indicates that bamboo strips were used to exorcise dead children.[37]

In China respect for parents (filial piety) who were deceased was displayed by the abstention of procreation, and more generally intercourse. Therefore, babies who were conceived during mourning were sometimes abandoned. Though during the Han dynasty taking the life of one's children was prohibited (unless it were born "deformed"), some parents may have justified the killing of an infant as delayed birth control, preventing the child from living a life of deprivation or suffering. There appeared to be ambivalence towards children due to the economic distress experienced by many families.

In ancient China, abandonment of infants was common, particularly after the birth of triplets, illegitimate birth, or if the child was born in the same month as the father. Newborns were left isolated, unfed and unnamed for three days after birth. The child and his or her mother were kept from the father for three months. If the father did not "lift up" and accepted the baby, he or she was abandoned. The rejected child was either exposed to the elements or was killed directly. Stillborn children were roasted or dismembered in order to eliminate a perceived dark spirit.[38]

To illustrate the extent to which female infanticide was performed in ancient China, the *Taipin jing,* a religious text which condemned the practice, states "Now under Heaven, all families kill girls; and under Heaven, how many hundreds of thousands of families are there? There are even some families that have killed more than ten girls." Of many reasons for killing baby girls was that parents had to pay out dowries upon their daughters' marriages. Other reasons were less practical: some texts such as *Sheng* ("Births") gave advice such as "whenever one gives birth on a *jisi* day, do not raise [the child]. It will be disadvantageous to its parents." Advice in these texts also included counsel against raising children who were born on the fifth day of the fifth month or with unusual physical characteristics.

Due to power struggles during early Imperial China, particularly during the Han and Qing dynasties, the killing of the emperor's children was fairly common, whether by the emperor himself or by those attempting to thwart the powers of the ruler. Empresses too would kill children of the emperor's concubines. In one example during the Han dynasty a long line of child murder began with Gaozu in 202 BC. The road to the throne was paved with the bodies of the emperors' sons (and their mothers) produced by his many concubines as well as his wife. The violence began when the empress killed the sons of the concubines in order to keep her own son and herself in power, as the favored sons of concubines could be put ahead of those born from the empress. In total, of the thirteen emperors of the Han dynasty, only three reigns were not tainted with child murder, although one of those three emperors attempted to murder his child unsuccessfully. Emperors, such as Chengdi, felt that they could always produce more sons, "a confidence that clearly figured in his decision to kill these infants"; consistent with the view of children in early China that children were replaceable and could be sacrificed for "greater glory of the patriline".[39]

The Buddhist religion stated that Nirvana was not available to those under the age of seven, thus a child's life was not valued until that point.[40] Because of this belief, Alexander the Great, during his conquests, noted widespread practice of infanticide in India. For example in the kingdom of Sophytes, who ruled along the Indus River, medical officers decided which children were to be raised and which were to be disposed of, based on defects real or imagined.[41]

One of the first efforts in the Eastern hemisphere to put an end to female infanticide was in 1789 by the British government. When the female population became so low as to be a burden, steps were taken to discontinue the practice. When men began to marry their own sisters and cousins due to the lack of females, or when the female population fell below twenty-five percent, female infanticide was discouraged.

Despite the widespread practice of infanticide, it was commonly believed among many societies that those not receiving a proper burial, children who died prematurely or victims of suicide, died what were deemed "a bad death" and the soul remained with the body; the younger the child at death, the greater the unused energy. This unused energy was said to be channeled into wrath or instability and thus induced more fear from the spirit of the child.[42]

Child Sacrifice in Ancient American Civilizations

Unlike other ancient civilizations, the Inca of Peru rarely practiced infanticide. Newborns were gifted land from the estates of those who had died, and twins were considered a gift from god as babies were considered a means to food and a livelihood. The Inca mostly sacrificed food, coca, animals, or figurines of people. When children were used, they were usually at least ten to twelve years old. One such child was found preserved in ice in the Andes, presumably as a gift to the mountain gods in order to bring various types of suitable weather. The frozen body of an approximately eight year old boy, who was found dressed in a camel wool poncho with several metal ornaments and figures, was also identified to have been from the Inca period. Another mummy of child, dated to about 5,000 years ago in Peru, was found elaborately prepared with a coat of clay and paint, and wrapped in a bird skin with a wig of human hair over the face. Some of the limbs were supported by sticks inserted under the skin. It is believed that perhaps the process of mummification indicates that the body was put on display for a time before interred.[43] Many other such mummies have been found in accessibly high funeral cairns. A sacrificed child of Incas would be strangled, bludgeoned or have his or her throat slit. It is hypothesized that the children were made to drink alcohol and were sacrificed by strangulation, or left in the mountains to die.[44] In addition to making an offer for good farming conditions, sacrifices were made to honor royalty. For example, for the coronation of a king two hundred children would be sacrificed. If an important person was ill, his son was sacrificed in hopes of appeasing the gods.[45]

Among the Olmecs of Mexico sacrifice of a fetus was performed to ensure rainfall. The human life cycle correlated to the life cycle of maize and the calendar. Similarly, the Guayaquil of Ecuador sacrificed one hundred children annually to appease the gods and to assure a good harvest. The Aztecs were particularly notorious for their tales of sacrifice. Human sacrifice was practiced for every Aztec festival where priests wore the victims' skins.[46] Children were drowned or decapitated to honor the rain god Tlaloc. At Temple Mayor a pit was unearthed which held the remains of children and infants. When a child was selected for sacrifice, he or she was indulged for a year; his or her only obligation was to play the flute. One the day of sacrifice the child's flute was smashed to signal the beginning of the ceremony.[47] While the Aztecs were criticized by the royal court for rampant child sacrifice, some religious intellectuals defended the practice by pointing to the Bible, in which infanticide had been acceptable in some cases.[48] Ironically, while most indigenous cultures in late civilizations killed or sacrificed deformed children, the Aztecs created institutions to care for them.[49] This is likely because the Aztecs deemed it a greater gift to use favored children. The Mayans also practiced sacrifice, but rather than using well-loved children, they purchased orphans or slaves, at a cost of five to ten stone beads. The child was either killed by cardiectomy or drowning. The ceremony took place on the top of a pyramid, and the child was painted blue and had his heart ripped out while it was still pulsating.

Vikings

The Vikings, too, practiced ritual sacrifice for the purpose of facilitating success in battle. One Viking chief killed his own seven year old son before heading off to war. Another reason for sacrifice would be to ensure a king's longevity. A Viking myth tells of King Aun, who at the age of sixty sacrificed his son to Odin, a major god of Norse mythology, who told the king that he would live forever if he gave him a son every ten years. After years of sacrificing nine of his sons he became bedridden and had to be carried around.[50]

Much like other ancient societies a Viking father would determine whether a newly born infant were to be kept or exposed. An exposure was called *utburd* (carrying out). When children were exposed, it was done non-violently. The infant would be securely placed in a covered grave, in a hallowed tree, or a between a hill of stones, so that no wild animal could get to it. A healthy baby who was abandoned, often for reasons of overwhelming poverty, discord between husband and wife, or superstition, was left with a piece of salt pork for it to suck on in case it was rescued by someone taking pity on it. Badly deformed infants were abandoned and buried out of fear, not malice, as it was believed these babies were born from evil. Once an accepted baby was baptized, exposure of an infant was considered murder if witnessed; however, a man could perform child sacrifice if done secretly.[51]

Bog bodies are considered a European phenomenon which represented sacrifice or punishment. Unlike the culturally created process of Egyptian mummification, bog bodies are preserved through the physical and chemical composition of bogs. One such "burial", which preserves the body because of microorganisms in the water, was of a mother and her newborn baby. Buried with the bodies was a pre-Roman clay vessel that was dated to the birth of Christ. Other children (and adults) have been found in these bogs without grave goods and with signs of extreme violence indicating not only evidence of sacrifice but punishment as well.[52]

Burial rituals among the ancients, while varied, tended to reflect the view that children were beloved, yet ephemeral. Eleanor Scott notes that at times, there was a tendency to interpret burials from the perspective of medieval, or later, views of parent-child relationships. Therefore, it is important to carefully consider the conclusions drawn by researchers within the multi-layered context in which they are deduced. The practice of burying newborns in the home, for example, is indicative of beliefs about the power of the dead over the living- the protection of siblings and the facilitation of fertility. It is also reflective of the fact neonates were not seen as full people, and therefore, did not require burial in consecrated ground. It is clear from the evidence left behind by the ancients that children were loved affectionately, but they were also often disposed of unceremoniously when deemed inconvenient, expensive, or excessive. While during this period, actions were taken to reduce infanticide and abandonment, many families chose whether or not to keep children based on the needs of their own families, and not the rules of the state.

4

Collateral of the Plague

Children of the Middle Ages and Renaissance

As the Middle Ages was a period of time marked by the plague, there was a remarkable decimation of the world population; a reduction from 450 million to about 350 million in the fourteenth century. In Europe alone the Black Death was estimated to have reduced the population from between thirty and sixty percent. As in other time periods, mortality among infants under the age of one year was high, and fifty percent of children did not make it to adult hood.[1] As a disproportionate number of children were felled by the plague, a greater appreciation of the very young manifested in the fourteenth and fifteenth centuries.[2]

Effects of the Black Death

The Black Death of the Middle Ages was actually three different types of plague. The fatal form, septicemic, was spread by fleas, while the pneumonic variety was spread by coughing and sneezing. The bubonic plague, also caused by fleas, was more widespread, representing seventy-five percent of all cases of the plague; however, it was less deadly and less contagious. Incidences of the bubonic plague tended to rise over spring and summer.[3] Because of misunderstandings of the nature of the different types of plague and the fear of contagion, the dead were often unceremoniously buried in pits.

While greater value was ascribed to children after the plague began to abate, some parents abandoned their children at the onset of the disease. Parents had no way of knowing the extent to which the pestilence would spread through a family. Children in particular were more likely to succumb to the disease, while the elderly were more likely to recover from certain strains of the plague. Greater immunity was acquired by exposure to various diseases during a life time; survival of one major epidemic increased the chances that one would survive another.[4] In 1363 a particular outbreak of plague killed mostly infants and toddlers, likely because it was the same strain to which older children and adults had already been exposed previously, and therefore, had acquired immunity.[5]

High mortality had a long lasting effect on the labor forces of Europe. In Tuscany in 1427 children and young adults up to age nineteen represented forty-four percent of the population, an unusually large percentage, while only forty-one percent of the population included productive adults. At this time children died before they could repay society the resources and energy devoted to them.[6] In addition, the lack of people available to perform labor increased wages as well as productivity. Historical economists believe that this facilitated the beginning of economic growth in Europe.

Although this book, and a great deal of the death literature, concerns itself with parent reactions to death, the discussion of children's responses to death, be it their own impending death or that of a sibling or friend, contributes to a fuller understanding of mourning in general, and the effects of an epidemic on the grieving process, specifically. A genre of children's literature which instructed in the practice of "the good" death presented itself in the form of seventeenth century texts for children titled *A Token for Children,* by James Janeway. This particular book included narratives of young children in Europe preceding their impending deaths. Two Dutch siblings, in particular, conducted themselves in such a singular manner, so near to their death, it has been proposed that they received both spiritual and emotional support from their parents, and that this support was distinctive for the time period. Their story was often reprinted as a model of "well-dying". The children, Susanna, aged thirteen, and Jacob, nine, lived in Lyden in 1664 where nearly 64,000 people perished from the plague the next year. The siblings also lost a younger sister to the disease. At the time, most people believed that the fatal form of the plague was spread through the air, rather than by fleas. Susanna was heard to ask "…is not God the Creator of the air? If it came out of the earth, is it not done by God?"[7] When sensing the end was near, Susanna begged her mother not to cry after her death, and for her father to comfort himself by channeling the biblical Job who lost all of his children but still said "The Lord has given, and the Lord has taken away, blessed be the name of the Lord".[8] Her little brother Jacob was equally steadfast. He parted with his toys and books stating: "…away with all my pleasant things in the world…"[9] It is clear that these children, fortified with religious teachings, loving parents, and entrenchment in a community greatly affected by the plague, learned not to fear death or suffer anxiety, but to accept their fate and comfort the living instead.

Abandonment and Infanticide in Medieval Europe

Children under the age of one represented sixty percent of all child deaths in medieval England. Most of these deaths were caused by fires and other accidents, as children were often left alone during harvest or while parents worked. In other instances, a very young infant left alone might choke on a sucking rag soaked in pap (an infant food of flour and milk or broth).

In medieval Europe abandonment and infanticide of infants was so prevalent that several foundling hospitals were established. In 1201 a legend illustrating the need for such hospitals, begins with Pope Innocent III, prompted by a vision, asking fishermen to cast nets into the Tiber River. Four hundred and twenty-seven drowned babies were retrieved from the river. On the basis of this tale, *Santo Spirito de Sassia* in Rome, a general hospital, opened a section for *expositi* (exposed or abandoned foundlings). Some foundling homes had a revolving door so that children could be left without humiliating and identifying parents. The first known foundling hospital, *Brephotrophia*, was established by the Byzantines in 400 AD for children, both abandoned and orphaned.[10] While the establishment of foundling hospitals or homes provided a solution to the widespread problem of infant abandonment (and subsequent death), these institutions had extremely high mortality rates (as discussed in Chapter 1). At Chartres, for example, mortality was an astonishing 100%. Crowding, disease, insufficient sustenance and wet nurses (and the pestilence carried by them) caused most children to die before the age of two.[11]

The crime of infanticide tended to reflect regional cultural biases. In Venice and England, for example, a mother's protestation of innocence was often accepted, whereas in other parts of Italy the mother was often met with suspicion when her child died. Illegitimate children in particular were susceptible to infanticide (discussed further in Chapter 11).[12] Infanticide, when identified as such, was punished by excommunication, and in some cities burning at the stake or beheading.

In response to widespread practice of murdering one's own children, San Bernardino, an associate of the Franciscan Fra Cherubino da Siena, was heard to say, "Go to Ponte Vecchio, there by the Arno, and put your ear to the ground and listen [to]…the voice of the innocent babies thrown into your Arno and your privies or buried alive in your gardens and your stables, to avoid the world's shame, and sometimes without baptism".[13]

It is often difficult to determine whether infanticide has been practiced, although gender ratios are one reliable method by which to determine whether deaths are a result of natural causes. Normal gender ratios are 105 to100 in favor of males. In fourteenth century England, for instance, the ratio of infants found was 133 to 100—given this great deviation from normal ratios one may deduce that those deaths were not a result of natural causes. In response to the widespread murder of children, myths were fabricated to cover the crime of infanticide with disappearance. *Kindlifresser*, an ogre who ate toddlers in Berne, Germany, was one such example. Similarly, Jews were accused of using the blood of Christian children for Passover rituals.[14]

In the *Yi li,* the Chinese book of etiquette and rites based on Confucianism, mourning rituals are described for children of different age groups. Parents of children, from the ages of three months to seven years, who had died were to wear no mourning clothes, and children younger than three months were "not to be wept for at all", although some texts state that for an infant under the age of three months, parents may weep one day for each day of the child's life. Evidence exists to show that many early Chinese, including emperors, disregarded these "rules", and grieved openly after elaborate funerals.[15]

Kinney asserts that the absence of funeral rites and burial practices for infants was a reflection of high mortality for very young children and thus a reticence of parents to become too attached; a theme that persists over and over in the child death literature. Materials found during archaeological excavations indicate that parents believed that the spirits of infants and children demanded attention after death. In some cases it was believed that frequent infant death in one family may suggest *Jie,* an attack on the family's living infants by the spirit of the deceased baby. In order to be rid of such spirits one could spray the bones of the deceased child with either dirt or ash.[16]

In Sung era China (907–1279 AD) children could be executed for striking a parent or grandparent. Among the poor, infanticide was common. If a man had numerous sons, he could have no more than four sons and three daughters.

A drowning bucket was kept near the birthing site to enforce this limitation. Eventually in 1659 Choen Tche made the first official edict against infanticide. Abandonment was also common among late-bearing parents whose estate had been divided up by first born children. Later in Hangchow, a foundling hospital was opened to take in these infants.[17]

The Crusades

The highly mythological and mysterious Children's Crusades are fraught with romanticism and tragedy. In 1212 a shepherd named Stephen began to speak of a children's crusade. As he travelled to Paris, reportedly many children followed him. While there is no real evidence of this event, and some writers have completely fictionalized this Crusade, there are other reports that children in Cologne moved across the Alps to get to Genoa, and then Rome. These 7,000 children were led by a boy named Nicholas. Many of the children were raped, and those who died were buried along the way. The trail turns cold when the children were supposedly on two boats that left for Pisa and were never seen again. There are no documents or personal histories from any of the hypothetical participants. Another group of children, numbering 30,000, were reported to have arrived in Marseilles. Sea captains provided seven ships to the children, two of which were lost in a storm. The bodies of the children supposedly washed up on the island of St. Peter, where Pope Gregory IX later built a church so that pilgrims could see the bodies (which inexplicably never decomposed). The remaining children were said to be sold as slaves in Egypt.[18] The lack of authoritative sources from the time of the Crusades, calls to question the authenticity of these stories. Nonetheless, children were casualties of these holy wars. During the first Crusade, for example, Jewish children were forced to commit suicide by and with their parents in order to avoid forced conversion to Christianity.[19]

Medieval Islam

Avner Gil'adi has written extensively on the bereavement of Muslim parents in the Middle Ages, and he refutes Philippe Aries' claim that parents did not suffer emotionally for the loss of their children. Due to recurring outbreaks of the Black Death, infant and child mortality was high in the Muslim world, as they were in other regions. And while the Black Death was never explicitly implicated in the consolation manuals written at this time, it is assumed that the plague was the cause of death for most Muslim children in the Middle Ages. For medieval Muslim parents in particular, consolation manuals were available in abundance—nearly thirty such books were published. These manuals illustrate the relationships between parents and children through evidence of their grief (See Chapter 9 for a discussion of consolation literature during this time). Although boys were favored for reasons beyond their ability to labor, female and male children alike were grieved at their death, and mortality did not appear to differ among socioeconomic classes. Gil'adi also notes that expressions of grief for a deceased child did not necessarily indicate a warm relationship.[20]

Some Muslim law experts believed that children should be honored as adults. For example, the body should be carried by people, not animals, and the preparation of the corpse and the prayer should be exactly the same as those for an adult. Many mourning rituals and reactions to death (not condoned by Islam) that were commonly practiced were often violent. These reactions included crying, screaming, moaning wailing, lamenting, "splitting collars", tearing off clothes, mutilating one's own face, shaving the head or tangling the hair, as well as reciting elegies and announcing one's death.[21] Additionally, some of the treatises spoke of parents who had died as a result of extreme reactions to grief. For example, a parent might refuse to eat or drink, sleep, or demonstrate complete apathy toward his or her own health. Avoiding these reactions was to inhabit the attribute of *sabr,* steadfastness. While the advice from the treatises appears to come from the time of Muhammed himself, the Prophet was noted to have very strong reactions to the deaths of his children and grandchildren. Thus a compromise is drawn, within these books, to accept emotional reaction in moderation.

While exhibiting *sabr* was thought to be rewarded, some demonstrations of steadfastness were unusual. Some parents were reported to have expressed happiness at their child's death. Some looked forward to the deaths of their children in the hope of "gaining otherworldly rewards for themselves…[some were known to] have encouraged their sons to sacrifice themselves, in a holy war, for instance"[22] Apparently it was believed that children who pre-deceased their parents would protect them from Hell and help them gain entry into Heaven. It is likely that these kinds of reactions to the death of a child are attributed to religious beliefs more so than a lack of parental affection.

Medieval Ireland

Children in Europe have always had special arrangements applied to their deaths. During the Middle Ages children were sewn into shrouds and buried in common graves.[23] Even in public cemeteries children were placed in special sections. For example, Jewish cemeteries in medieval Winchester and York had a separate plot for children. In Ireland, however, *cillini,* burial grounds for children (also discussed in the context of prehistoric Ireland in Chapter 2), were reserved primarily for unbaptized infants as well as other individuals deemed unsuitable for burial in consecrated ground, such as the mentally ill, criminals, strangers, and famine and suicide victims. Historians and archaeologists date the inception of the latter context of these burials grounds anywhere from the early medieval period to the nineteenth century. It is believed that their development was in connection to reinvigorated Catholicism in Ireland. Locations of the *cillini* were places such as deserted churches or graveyards, ancient monuments, or natural landmarks. Usually there was no fence and many were built near forts. Some of the children were found buried with grave goods such as several pebbles and a stone anthropogenic figurine; perhaps a doll for the child to take with him to the afterlife. Additionally, it was customary to leave a handful of quartz pebbles and one long stone pebble in each grave of a newborn. The pebbles had two functions: first, quartz has been used as a decorative item since prehistoric days, and second, it was believed to have had protective properties (and was a Christian practice), conferring a religious dimension to burials denied a consecrated burial.[24] Some children were buried in Scots Pine coffins, while others, especially stillborn or newborn infants, were shrouded. These graves were often simply marked, albeit rudimentarily and without inscription as only the wealthy would be able to afford headstones made of anything better than wood or rocks.[25]

Cillini came to exist as the Church of England forbade unbaptized children to be buried within consecrated ground. In Hereford Cathedral, for example, walls were built to prohibit the burial of unbaptized infants as sometimes midwives would be paid to bury a stillborn child that they had delivered. Baptism of the newly born could often be problematic. In a time where infant death was common, baptisms were often performed within the first week of life. In medieval London midwives were given the authority to baptize dying newborns lest they die in a state of original sin. If a mother were to die in childbirth, a midwife was instructed to cut the child from the womb and baptize it —but only if a man were not immediately available.[26] If the death of an infant appeared probable baptism could take place when the head emerged. If a hand or foot was delivered first, the limb could be baptized and the full sacrament could be administered after the birth, if the baby survived.[27]

Irish folklore exists in which dead children transformed into changelings or murderesses. These stories have associations with *cillini,* and other similar sites, and have contributed to the preservation of these sites due to the superstitions. Additionally, Finlay asserts that the marginal location, and "the character of these sites and the type of burial deposits does not encourage visitation as an active act of remembrance. Folklore evidence and testimony on the use of the sites confirms the discreet nature of the burial."[28] Murphy, on the other hand, argues that while the Church may have excluded these babies from commemoration, this did not preclude parents from grieving. The selection of these sites which were prominent, yet in disrepair and likely to be left undisturbed but not forgotten, indicates that the burials were not marginal. Additionally, these sites often had an earlier religious function making them an optimal alternative to consecrated burial in light of their former sanctity and physical protection. These discreet and liminal types of burials are often interpreted as depositories for victims of infanticide; however, unwanted babies would have been treated as refuse and not placed in a protected environment with symbolic religious meaning. Murphy also argues that the selection of poor land near marshes or bogs would have been a good choice to allow for dead family members to remain undisturbed. Since most peasants did not own their own land, it is unlikely that the landowners would allow usable agricultural land for *cillini.*[29]

Many parents were distressed at their inability to bury their children in consecrated ground. A woman by the name of Mrs. Salmon, on her eightieth birthday, received a lifelong wish when the Church blessed two of her dead children who had been refused a church burial. In a similar vein, a priest affected by the plight of grieving parents blessed a plot of land by the sea that held the remains of one hundred unbaptized neonates.[30]

With respect to burials in medieval Ireland, usually it was the father or other men in the family that would bury the child at night with little commemoration. For a funeral for a newborn baby the family might have viewed it from afar, while the father and a neighbor buried the infant. When infants died during or shortly after birth, medieval mothers often had a fairly extended laying in period (as much as two weeks), and often found themselves unable to attend the funeral.[31]

The Renaissance

During the Renaissance in Italy, people were preoccupied with death. Depictions of death could be found everywhere: in poetry, art, and on tombs. Of the thousands, if not millions, of children who died during the Middle Ages, Margaret King writes of the privileged Valerio Marcello, an eight year old boy who's death in 1461 sent his father into inconsolable despair. Jacopo Antonio Marcello of Venice was a nobleman, an active military man and soldier, as well as a patron of the arts and humanities. Despite the fact that he was able to perform his duties dependably, as a public figure he was admonished by his peers for his inability to relinquish his grief. The senior Marcello contributed a compilation of the works addressed to him by poets, writers, historians, and friends, which he had illustrated in gilt, to the consolation literature of the Renaissance period. Although never completed, this collection of poetry, letters, eulogies, and apologies represents the largest and most resonant consolatory collection of the Renaissance.[32]

During the Renaissance, monuments to the dead were widespread in Europe, with the majority erected for adults. If children were commemorated at all, then it was most often within the context of the monument for the adult. In Renaissance era Poland, however, funeral monuments for children were prevalent. Jeannie Labno cataloged forty-four funerary monuments constructed for children, of 333 total monuments built for children. This collection included monuments for both girls and boys, and appears to be a strong indicator of attitudes toward children as well as gender. The monuments were dated to the early sixteenth century. Most monuments included a motif of a *putto* and a skull. The sleeping *putto* (like a little angel) references the infant Jesus in depictions of the Virgin and child. The appeal "to [the] commonly understood emotion of motherly love enabled bringing the mourners closer to God", and helped the family come to terms with the death.[33] Of Labno's research, one of the most famous examples is a monument to three stillborn babies, possibly the children of the mayor of Olawa, Poland. In fact, most of the monuments are to the very young -under age three. Some monuments also depicted children lovingly embracing their parents, illustrating sentiments of familial bonds.

The Laments of Jan Kochanowski , a great poet of Poland (whose poetry is discussed in more detail in Chapter 9) are commonly abstracted or adapted on inscriptions of monuments in Poland. Kochanowski's own Laments were written after the death of his two year old daughter. One particularly moving inscription, written by Kochanowski for another family (and subsequently adapted) is as follows:

> Here lies Piotr Mikolaj Karczewski his parent's affection, Or more aptly his tears and his lamentation...A gracious delightful, uncommonly talented child/who having shown great tokens of all youthful virtues/suddenly, and without warning passed away/in his unripe years,/to the great and unbearable sorrow of his parents/ written with tears by Jan Karczewski, his unhappy father,/for his dearest son/...He did not stay long on this earth twenty weeks. He was born on Monday in April and gave his breath to God on Thursday [the festival of the Holy Cross] in the year 1601[34]

Monuments were considered a replacement for the "Social Body" of the deceased; their role in society and family, and their achievement as evidenced by the size, location, heraldry and materials used. Thus, attitudes toward death and burial rites impacted the commemorative practices of later societies. Compared to Poland, other European societies did not regard the child as highly. This too, suggests familial relations were different in Poland than elsewhere. It is worth noting that although some societies may not regard children highly, it does not speak to personal reactions to a death. Children were viewed from the perspective of the potential they held as future adults, a phenomenon seen among prehistoric families as well, where children were buried with tools that they may have used in the future. Further, children were seen as a sign of God's blessing or a symbol of dynastic achievement. "Erecting a funeral monument to a child accords a child a second burial."[35]

Noble Children of the Renaissance

The nobility of the Renaissance period received unusual treatment in death. Among the dynastic rulers of Europe, baptized infants would be buried in church yards, while other family members would not. Excarnation, the removal of flesh and organs, was common performed among adult nobility, the Hapsburgs in the nineteenth century in particular. The procedure, however, was not performed on children. Instead, noble children were eviscerated (removal of entrails).[36] Organs of six noble children were found buried in urns at St. Stephens. Burials at night were not only relegated to common or poor children. With the exception of an heir to the throne, burial ceremonies for children under the age of twelve were often clandestine. Children were often buried close to the place of death. Further, every effort was made to baptize a dying child. For example, a six month old fetus was cut out of the dead empress Maria Anna of Spain, and baptized before it died in 1646.

With the advent of high child mortality caused by neglect, accidents, and the plague, we are able to see how the society at large suffered from a reduction in the labor force, and how parents appeared to mourn their children in conformity to religious expectations; whether with the steadfastness expected of Muslim parents, or with the haste made to baptize newborns lest they wander in purgatory forever. Parents may have been used to losing children, babies in particular, but with the Black Death they were losing them in quick succession and often all at once. Additionally, one is able to observe that quite often mourning rituals and the cultural conditions facilitating infanticide remained rather static from ancient history to the Middle Ages; China is one notable example. Religious institutions, in particular, attempted to reduce the gross acts of infanticide taking place. In the late Middle Ages and in the Renaissance we began to see a resurgence is the idolization of the child, particularly in Poland, and particularly in artwork (as will be discussed in Chapter 10).

5

Ambivalence, Christianity, Slavery, and the Devil

America and England in the 17th to 20th Centuries

After the first Boston small pox epidemic in 1677 when thousands of children died, parents were cautioned to restrain affection to their children so as not to become too attached to them. Therefore, fear of childhood death facilitated the aloof nature of parent-child relationships at this time. In the early 1800s children began to be thought of as innocents, changing not only childhood experiences, but the way children were treated at death.[1]

The 1800s also marked a turn in mothers' behavior in colonial America, which included bonding with their children. Just fifty years prior, a culture of ambivalence appeared to limit parental concern for American children. In fact, some historians regard parental responses to child death as evidence of self-control rather than ambivalence. Religious belief played a large part in demonstrating steadfastness, as it was often believed that the life of the child was the responsibility of God. While records, such as diaries, from this time note that parents appeared to accept child death as an expected milestone of life, other accounts demonstrate that parents despaired at the illnesses or deaths of their children.

Divine Providence

The Puritan minister and scholar, Cotton Mather, was once heard to explain that his daughter being badly burned in a fire was a punishment for his own sin. Expanding on this example, it would seem that relying on Divine Providence, the mercurial protector of children, seemed to preclude colonial parents from paying attention to their children's health and safety needs.[2] Parents often gave themselves up to the belief that their children would be taken away from them for the benefit of god.

To further reflect this deference to God in matters of a child's life and death, Louisa Park in 1801 exclaimed, after the death of her beloved infant son, "Yet I do not wish thee back again, my lovely innocent. No—I will bless my God who has taken thee to Himself before though couldst offend him, and has saved thee from a life of sickness, sorrow, and woe, although it has been at the expense of my health and happiness." It is as though parents comforted themselves with the idea that children were better off dead and in heaven.[3]

Responsibility for Child Mortality

In nineteenth century America the mortality rate of children under the age of five represented forty percent of the total death rate. As the mortality rate began to climb, due to urbanization (infant mortality was recorded as 235 per 1000 in the year 1900, although inaccurate birth records render these numbers imprecise), women began to change their attitudes toward responsibility for their children's welfare; a responsibility that caused much anxiety. Given the high mortality rate, women's writings suggested that "the experience of infant death formed a constant backdrop against which mothers' experiences and emotions must be set".[4] Later, as sanitary conditions and nutrition improved, and infant mortality declined, women's responses to their families, again, changed. While in colonial America the community helped to care for children, although "Divine Providence" was employed to explain infant death, by the beginning of the nineteenth century the belief that the mother was responsible for the welfare of the child became widely accepted. Women, working through social welfare and reform groups, began to voice their concerns over the high mortality rates of their children. The shift to making infant mortality the concern of the public, government bureaucracies, and health professionals created a culture of shared responsibility for all children.[5]

Despite the shared responsibility for the welfare of the young, infant death became a private matter as concern for children left God's hands and entered the mother's. As long as mothers were aware that children did not need to die, women did not need to resign themselves to a lifetime of mourning over children. Rather, they could employ newly found knowledge about childcare and sanitation in order to improve their children's chances of survival.[6] Mothers knew, however, that their actions alone could not create the conditions necessary within their communities to keep their babies healthy. In the early twentieth century, spurred by social reformers, mothers fought for adequate sanitation, clean water and pure milk, as well as education on childbirth and infant care. Mothers were well aware that their children had been sacrificed by their ignorance. The Federal Children's Bureau, established in 1912, received letters from mother's across the country asking for assistance in the matters of keeping their families alive. For example, although the Naval Academy Dairy pasteurized milk and made ice daily, none of it was available for sale to the surrounding community. The government's indifference toward children's well-being was reflected in the frustration of these mothers.[7]

Colonial and Victorian Era Grief

While few records exist from the early colonial period, those examined by historians, in the form of diaries and autobiographies, indicated expressions of grief. Smart argues that many of the records that were left behind from the colonial American era were written by men, and therefore, only express the male point of view. Fathers were often steadfast in their grieving and admonished mothers for their public displays of mourning. The following examples, however, illustrate how fathers were not always stoic in the face of a child's death. For example, one father wrote upon the death of his four year old daughter "The grief for this child was so great that I forgot myself so much that I did offend God in it…I …could not be comforted, although my friends spoke so comfortably to me."[8] In another example, William Palfrey writes in 1772 of his seven year old daughter "…I go about crying like a fool whenever I think of her".[9]

Despite the above examples, the great majority of writing on grief demonstrates resignation to God's will. Dye and Smith present the diary of a mother of twelve children, eight of whom died as infants, who describes her daughter's death in these terse terms "Sept 9 It died about 8 o'clock in the morning… Sept 10 Was buried." This account has been often quoted as an example of not only resignation to God's will, but the demonstration of "due distance" from a child.[10] The Puritan Thomas Skinner warned parents not to get too attached to their children as they may leave you "sighing and desolate".[11] Even when parents did not heed this advice, Puritan children were seen as wicked and depraved. Salvation was not available for Puritans; therefore, there was no comfort for parents that their children would rest in heaven, although clergymen would imply to grieving parents that the child's soul would be saved. Nonetheless, parents were advised to grieve with self-control. The Virginia Gentry too were advised to temper their mourning with the comforting thought that another child might come to replace the one lost.[12]

Women's Writings

Because most texts on grief in early Colonial America were written by men, Dye and Smith have postulated whether the lack of women's writings can be interpreted as an acknowledgement that until an infant grew into a healthy child they were not yet considered a full person, and thus his or her well-being was not in control of the mother. As more children began to survive their infancy, writings by mothers more fully described the lives of their children. These works indicated, perhaps, the willingness of mothers to spare more emotion for children that were more likely to stay.[13] Accordingly, once mortality rates dropped, sentimentality began to return to the parent-child literature of the time. At this time fiction and poetry in popular periodicals exhorted the idea that the death of a child was part of God's plan to enable the family to reunite in heaven.[14]

Grieving Victorian Mothers

Women in the Victorian Era were often perceived as weak and perhaps well-suited for expressing grief. The consolation literature of this time included prayers, poetry, songs and stories written to comfort grieving families. Thus, it became acceptable for women to grieve openly. Another means of mourning was in the creation of mourning quilts. Making the quilt allowed women to grieve and also leave a memorial. The practice was particularly salient among those who were not literate enough to enjoy the benefit of the consolation literature that was so popular at the time.[15] Other expressions of grief included photographs, and artwork (discussed further in Chapter 10), as well as fashioning hair jewelry (from the hair of the deceased).

Treatment of the Stillborn

The lack of documentation of stillbirths in history is a limitation of demographic research. Some researchers postulate that this lack of recording is indicative of attitudes toward neonates. Many disposed stillborn children were found buried in very shallow graves in marginal areas. The nature of these burials allows for the resting places to be disturbed by land developers and scavenging animals. In Scotland the body of a stillborn child was easily disposed of. Often Scottish children, who died within twenty-four hours of birth, were submitted to undertakers to be buried as a stillborn because the burial was cheap, quick, and did not require a funeral service. Some unscrupulous funeral directors would falsify burial certificates in order to save the reputation of a mother who had given birth to an illegitimate child. By noting that a child was stillborn, when in fact the child died soon after birth, would relieve any speculation of infanticide (even if the mother had indeed killed her newborn). Single mothers who gave birth to living children, who soon died, were often accused of infanticide. Additionally, sometimes, in order to save money, two bodies were buried in one coffin. The lack of government regulation over births facilitated these practices, and caused a significant underreporting of births, and gross acts of covering up infanticide. In order to mitigate the effects of similar behaviors in their countries, both France and England adopted systems of requiring birth registration within three days of a baby's arrival. Single women in particular did not wish to see their "mistakes" or "sins" registered in the public record. The Registration of Still-Births Act in Scotland came to pass in 1939, which required that a doctor or midwife provide a cause of death on the death certificate of any stillborn child after the 28th week of gestation. This act subsequently raised the status of neonates during the early 20th century.[16]

Grave Stones, Epitaphs, and Burials

Michelle Vovelle, studying Epitaphs found on American gravestones, points out that with the surge of deaths of young children and mothers around the year 1780 the function of the epitaph changed from a "perpetuation of honors… [to] an expression of family grief". Further, the text of the epitaph itself clarified the manner in which Americans perceived death and the afterlife. For example, in the mid-1700s, twenty percent of epitaphs were written in Latin, while less than a century later only two percent were. This shift illustrates the move from formal inscriptions to more personal commemorations.[17]

Additionally, the use of euphemisms for death such as "fell asleep" or "departed this life" indicates an aversion to a direct reference to the dead body. Vovelle counted at least fifty such metaphors for death on gravestones. Conversely, there was an increase in the details used to describe causes of death. On the gravestones of the young the circumstances of their demise were not only noted, but commented upon. For example, one epitaph, written by the parents of children who froze to death when their ship was run aground after a trip around the world, implored, "And now Lord God Almighty, just and true are all Thy ways, but who can stand before Thy cold?"[18] Epitaphs such as these also signify the move toward mourning openly for family members. For example, Cotton Mather, the Puritan minister well known for his involvement in the Salem Witch Trials, buried his unbaptized four day old son under the epitaph, "Reserved for a Glorious Resurrection".[19]

During westward expansion in America, families on wagon trains had to bury their children wherever the death occurred along the long journey. In one case, the parents of a child who was killed by a stampede left a note for other travelers to tend to the grave. Upon return, fellow travelers of the grieving family noted that not only was the grave tended but a log fence was built around it for protection.[20]

Slave Children

The brutal Middle Passage journey from Africa to the Caribbean, as well as the physical demands of working on plantations, while taxing on adult slaves, was particularly lethal for slave children. From 1813 to 1816 about one half of slave children lived to the age of five. The primary causes of death were insufficient food, illness from unclean conditions, and infection at birth from unsanitary practices.[21]

As slave reformers campaigned for better conditions, infant and child mortality rates decreased. The relationship between these two factors, however, may not be linear as it is uncertain whether plantation owners heeded reformers. Slave owners varied in their treatment of slave children. Some reduced workloads for pregnant and nursing women with rewards for bearing and raising living children, while many others continued to treat all slaves equally cruelly. Preferential treatment of pregnant or nursing mothers appeared to characterize the time period after the abolition of the British slave trade in 1807. While the slave population grew from the 1820s to 1830s, on some plantations the birth rate in general was low. Infertility was caused by physical stress and poor diet. Additionally, slave women, wishing to save their unborn children from similar oppression, would eat dirt or other substances to induce miscarriages; others poisoned their newly born infants. Some scholars have interpreted the high rate of miscarriages as an attempt on the part of slave women to stay attractive and shapely in order to attract the attention of white males who could improve their social status.[22]

The high mortality rate for slave children in particular is explained not only by physical abuse and hazardous working conditions, but also by poor nutrition. The slave diet in general was lacking in proteins that contained the eight essential amino acids. Cornmeal and fatty meats, like pork, were the staple food items provided by slave owners. Pregnant and nursing mothers, already deficient in the minerals necessary for their own good health, were unable to properly nourish growing fetuses, which would rely on the maternal store of minerals if her diet was insufficient. Subsequent pregnancies would diminish the maternal store even further, leaving a fetus undernourished before it was even born. Breastfeeding only perpetuated these mineral deficiencies for both mother and child. While weaning a child to a "full diet" would have provided the necessary respite for the mother and an opportunity for the baby to get the minerals needed, the diet the child was weaned to was even less sufficient. Plantation owners felt that vegetables and lean meats and were not good for children. Thus, children's diets consisted of cornbread, hominy, and fat. Cow's milk might have mitigated some of the effects of this poor regimen, but this too, was withheld from slave children. Additionally, vitamin D, if not available in the diet, could be absorbed through the skin by exposure to sunlight; however, the dark skin of Africans, meant to keep the skin cool and provide protection from the sun, also inhibited the absorption of the vitamin to some degree.[23]

Malnourishment led children to become susceptible to a great deal of illnesses. Fifty-one percent of all slave deaths were children under the age of nine, while white children accounted for thirty-eight percent. The six causes of death to which slave children were most susceptible were convulsion, teething, tetanus, lockjaw, suffocation, and worms. Teething was attributed as a cause of death because it was often a precursor to hasty weaning. In a slave child's diet breast milk was often the only source of calcium ever available to him. The direct cause of death in these cases was tetany, a severe twitching of the muscles, which is caused by a lack of calcium.

Smothering was also disproportionately attributed as a cause of death to slave children. For example, of the 723 suffocation deaths in the year 1849, ninety-two percent were black infants. In retrospect, it appears that Sudden Infant Death Syndrome (SIDS) might have been the direct cause of death. Parents may have thought that they had "overlain" or unintentionally smothered an infant in the night, and thus caused their death. Many of the indicators for SIDS babies in modern times were also present in slave babies. These indicators include low birth weight and respiratory illness.[24]

Burial Practices for Slave Children

Most of the inherited cultural practices of their ancestors were denied to slaves in America, with the exception of mortuary behavior. While slave owners would have controlled nearly every aspect of slave life, some practices, specifically burying their own dead, were "permitted". In comparing slave cemeteries to burial sites in Africa, Jamieson provides evidence that funerary practices were carried over from Africa. While rare today, New World slave mortuary practices were widespread; although, cultural transmission of mortuary behavior is strong in general among many groups. Church burials were denied to slaves as they were not baptized Christians. So, slaves were left by whites to bury the dead within their own cemeteries, with special groups of slaves to prepare the body. Funerals in New York, for example, were the only times slaves could gather in groups larger than three.[25] Characteristics of slave burials included mounds of 1/2m -1 m high, with burials in and around the mounds. Grave goods were either sentimental or an item that would serve the deceased after death. Some African groups buried all of the deceased's possessions in the grave. It was believed that the grave good belonged only to the living, and was buried with the deceased in order to get the trapped soul out of grave.[26] For the funeral of the infant son of an African born slave in the 1830s, for example, the child was buried with a small bow and arrow and a miniature canoe in order to help him cross the ocean to his own country. The child was also buried in white muslin with figures painted on it so that the father's countrymen would know the infant to be his son.[27]

There are other mortuary rituals practiced by American slaves which also had been carried over from African cultures. In Ghana, for example, there were separate burials for different social groups which were often tied to the cosmology of the group; those who died of natural causes were distinguished from those who did not. People who died a natural death were buried within the house, while among the Yoruba, for example, those who did not were buried out of town. Burial places were often related to the cause of death; drowning victims were buried at the river bank where they died, while infants were buried behind the mother's hut. Empty marked graves indicated those who had died who couldn't be brought back for burial. Dead children among the Ghanaian tribes were buried separately at a crossroads. Among the Asante, children under eight days old were buried in pots in town. Family burials in one grave were also common.

Newsboys

Children who died during the nineteenth century were generally buried by family, the church, or the cultural group to which they belonged. DiGirolamo brings to light the practices of newsboy funerals in which other young colleagues, sometimes orphans and homeless themselves, but certainly always poor, laid their peers to rest. Newsboys often collected money for coffins and headstones, the minister, and flowers. They also participated in public funeral processions through the streets in which they lived and worked. While obscure, and usually occurring in major U.S. cities such as New York, Boston, Philadelphia, and Chicago, these practices were unusual given the public sphere in which they took place. Further, parentless boys did not die unloved and alone. Indeed the newsboys considered each other family, and the elaborate manner in which these children in poverty were buried and mourned further demonstrates the esteem in which they held each other.[28]

If indifference to the regular occurrence of children dying was the assumed rule, then the case of newsboys was the exception. Newsboys were often the subject of consolation literature, which included sermons, poems, memories, and other writings. Poems include Emily Thornton's "The Dying Newsboy" (1886) and Irene Abbott's "Only a Little Newsboy" (1903), which appeared in popular magazines. These poets were less concerned about exposing social conditions, and more about moving readers to help the poorest of children. Poets and those who helped the newsboys, their employers and ministers for example, found their cause an opportunity for "moral instruction."[29]

The question of how to appropriately bury poor children was a common problem, as funerals were (and still are) expensive. Among the poor working class in the nineteenth century it was not uncommon to find deceased infants buried in anonymous graves or abandoned in the streets. Jacob Riis noted that seventy-two deceased (from natural causes) babies were picked up in 1890s New York alone. The bodies of these infants were most likely abandoned because parents could not afford their funerals, although older children were usually properly buried. Funerals for children could impoverish families for weeks. Funerals for older children, who were often more likely afforded a funeral than a baby, were much more costly.

Lou Taylor noted that when the body of a child was too long to fit under the seat of the hearse driver, the cost of the funeral went up.[30]

In addition to paying for a coffin, flowers, the burial and service, newsboys also published resolutions in order to publicly express their condolences, whether for a public figure or for one of their colleagues. While children, prior to the twenty-first century, grew up to be with death (whether experienced in their own families or through sermons at church), newsboys' experiences with death were even more sophisticated given the location of their "offices". Many were witness to the funeral processions of the most famous and revered public figures like President Lincoln. When Ulysses S. Grant died, several hundred boys went to city hall to state the fact of their sympathy for the passing of the president. They felt it was "our privilege to give expressions of regret and sympathy so universal". They then insisted that the resolution be sent to Grant's children and wife, who later acknowledged the consolation. A similar resolution was written for a fellow newsboy, which included "Whereas, Willie Crawford was a good fellow…he was always square and honest…he should have lived longer…it is no more than right to let his mother know what a good fellow he was when he was with us…." The newsboys also wrote obituaries, submitting them to the newspapers for which they worked. Often these obituaries mirrored their resolutions; a mention of the deceased's qualities, the circumstances by which he died, and the regret for the bad hand of cards the boy was dealt. Newsboys were elaborate in their expressions of sorrow; while excessive grieving was generally looked down upon, the newsboys would sob and sing during funeral processions.[31]

Because elaborate funerals with all of the trimmings indicated an elevated status, as well as an expression of deep affection, the boys went all out when they could. For one boy in particular, a cortege, reserved for male funerals only, of fifty-six boys, six of them pall bearers, led a procession from the boy's home to the church, passing the child's newsstand. Alexander Hogeland, who founded the Newsboys' and Bootblacks' association in Louisville, noted that he was often the only adult to attend these funerals in addition to the undertaker and parent. For a funeral procession the coffin would be draped in black crepe, with a white ribbon that symbolized that the coffin held a child.

It was the fear of a potter's field, which concerned these boys. To them the quality of their graves and funerals had a direct relationship to the "condition" of their soul. Burial in potter's field was an everlasting indignity. The elaborate funerals, obituaries, and mourning rituals were a way of articulating that they were humans and tradesmen and not nameless vagrants.[32] "Respectability, to them, was taking care of their own, which somehow became more important in death than in life." The fear of being buried in a potter's field prompted some boys to take advantage of burial clubs or insurance companies so that they would be afforded the elaborate funeral they deserved. Newspapers, at times, helped to cover the costs of a newsboy's funeral. It was not in the name of self-promotion either, as competing periodicals reported the kind acts.[33]

Funerals and Mourning Dress in the Nineteenth Century

Small circular hearses were used to transport the dead in the late nineteenth century. White hearses, as well as white clothes, were intended only for children—symbolizing innocence and purity. Only the grieving wore black. Wealthier families, who could afford it, also adorned all accessories in white: white gloves, scarves, ostrich feathers for the black horses, and white saddle fittings. Children, when parents could afford it, were memorialized in the same manner as adults. When young unmarried girls died, it was not uncommon for the services to mirror that of weddings with bridal wreaths adorning the church or the girl's coffin. A betrothed, if not yet married, girl might be dressed in her wedding gown. The purpose of these ceremonies was to attempt to deceive sprits into believing that the unmarried had in fact been wed.[34]

In some cultures mourning is very specifically prescribed. For example, in nineteenth century Korea, in addition to the instructions for mourning dress and sacrifice, parents and grandparents are expected to mourn children (who are also divided into age classes) one degree less than for adults. For those under eight years of age no mourning garments are worn, and for a baby under three months "there is not even wailing". If a child is betrothed, despite his or her age, mourning is worn as though for an adult.[35]

Causes of Death in Nineteenth Century England

To illustrate the nature of child death and community response in the nineteenth century, Sambrook investigated a sample of constabulary letters, reports written by police officers on the day of the child's death and given to the coroner, in Staffordshire, England from 1851 to 1860. These letters described the sudden deaths of 6,000 children ranging in age from newborn to twelve years of age. Twelve percent of the deaths were related to work (for the older children), while the remainder occurred in or around the home. The most common causes of death were accidental burns and drowning. Most of the children who died from scalding or burning were between two and three years of age. Half of all of these cases occurred when the parents were either at work or, more frequently, while the mother was on an errand.[36]

Often the community could be counted on to come to the assistance of a child in a crisis, or to support a grieving parent. While "the public voice", as it was referred to, could be called upon to inform authorities about poor treatment of a child, it did not protest the practice of leaving young children alone while their parents were at work. Frequently, children as young as six years of age could be found caring for infants. Many times multiple families of children would be left together to care for each other; establishing a dangerous, yet widely accepted, "child care" practice. Even though these child care arrangements were accepted by families and their neighbors, the authorities were also aware of the extent of the neglect. Police officers admonished mothers for putting their children's lives at risk for the price of their income. It was not until 1899 when the Poor Law Guardians were empowered to take children from unsuitable parents.[37]

As mentioned in Chapter 1, the practice of insuring one's child against death, injury, or illness raised suspicion of foul play, especially when one family experienced repeated tragedies. In the Black Country, England, death clubs paid fifty shillings to a parent upon the death of a child. In the cases where death clubs were employed, suspicious police officers took note of a possible motive for child murder, such as whether the dead child was illegitimate. Of the 594 cases where parents received a death benefit, eight percent of the children were illegitimate; the illegitimacy rate of the entire population averaged about six percent during this time.

Sambrook notes that it is difficult to ascertain the collective emotions of the grieving parents of Staffordshire, as the police who took the reports did not record that type of information in their reports. She postulates that it is entirely reasonable that while by today's standards parents may have been neglectful or careless, they still could have been anguished at the time of their child's death. This granular detail would have provided more insight into the grief patterns during this time period, and whether death was intentional (e.g., in order to collect death club payouts) if they had been included in constabulary reports—even if the information is subjectively observed. What was been noted in the reports, however, is that police officers would ascertain from neighbors comments whether or not a child had been treated kindly during his or her life. This information is helpful in determining the extent of concern for children, whether dead or alive.[38]

Accusations of Infanticide

Women accused of murdering their newborn babies were tried under the 1624 Act to Prevent the Destroying and Murdering of Bastard Children. However, treatment of these mothers changed in London, from 1674 to 1803. Historian Mary Clayton analyzed these changes via the Old Bailey trials of England. For example, the "childbed linen" defense was first used in 1689 by Mary Campion. This defense stated that the mother had, in fact, prepared for the birth of her child, and therefore, it was wanted and its death unintentional.[39]

Likewise, Caron investigated the changing attitude of medical professionals toward infanticide cases in Providence, Rhode Island from 1870 to 1938. During this time, doctors began to legitimize the defense of postpartum insanity as a cause of infanticide. This defense was often used among women who gave birth alone; a difficult and disorienting endeavor. Some factors that pointed to guilt, with respect to intentional infanticide, were the lack of preparation for the impending birth, violence to the infant's body, or evidence of strangulation. Hydrostatic tests could also be used to prove guilt. With a hydrostatic test the lungs are removed from a child thought to be a victim of infanticide. The organs are then placed on the surface of distilled water. If the lungs sink, then there is no evidence that the child ever breathed, and therefore, it is unlikely that it was killed after birth. The procedure is controversial in that decomposition of the body could cause gases to accumulate in the lungs without the infant breathing, causing the lungs to sink-incorrectly signifying murder. Many people, including doctors who could not fathom killing one's own flesh and blood, were also willing to reason that no lucid mother would kill her child, thus making a case for temporary insanity. During this particular time period in Rhode Island the infanticide rate had actually decreased, which is attributed, in part to the opening of a the *Sophia Little Home* for unwed mothers and their babies. Additionally, abortion became a crime in 1861. A campaign for the consideration of the importance of the unborn child may have mitigated situations where women considered infanticide.[40]

In light of options for women with regard to unwanted or inconvenient babies, Burnston attempts to explain what she describes as the abnormal behavior related to the placement of two infants found in a "privy pit" of a wealthy home. One infant was dated from 1750–65 the other 1780–85. There are several possible explanations for these findings, but none are satisfactory. Burnston refutes the arguments that children who died of natural causes were discarded in the trash because it was too expensive for poor women to bury them properly; charity funerals were always an option. Further, during the eighteenth century fear of contagion of yellow fever might preclude anyone from disposing of even a tiny infected corpse in the communal garbage. Poor women might have abandoned a bastard child; a wealthy woman pregnant with a "bastard" child might have paid someone else to care for it, or she might have gone away at the beginning of her pregnancy and returned without the child.[41] Despite all of these apparently logical reasons for burying a dead child properly, or avoiding killing an unwanted child, it is likely that a desperate or mentally ill person, who committed the irrational and unfeeling act of putting a baby in a toilet, cannot be puzzled out so easily, if at all.

During the late eighteenth and nineteenth centuries many changes in behaviors and perceptions could be noted. Prior to the Industrial Revolution a shift in women's attitudes toward children and child death was observed. Previously, Divine Providence or "god's will" could be blamed for a child's death. As responsibility for the survival of the young shifted to parents, and mothers in particular, grief became a more private affair. Further, as positive changes in public health policy induced lower mortality rates, women's relationships with their children began to change. Further, women worked harder to ensure that their children survived. Diaries left behind from the colonial and Victorian Eras are contradictory; some show evidence of debilitating grief, while others demonstrate resignation to frequent child death. Burial practices, too, began to shift. While the burial of slave children tended to reflect the practices of African cultures, epitaphs on colonial tombstones demonstrated an evolution towards more personalization. Further, laws pertaining to infanticide protected both the accused and young victims, although neglect and illegitimacy were still major factors contributing to both natural deaths and infanticide, respectively.

6 Modern Times

The Psychology of Grief

At present, on the internet one can find instructions on how to do anything, from making a bomb to baking a chocolate soufflé, from how to potty train your child to how to mourn your child. Wikihow.com, for example, has a twenty-five step process on how to "Survive the Death of your Child (with Pictures)". While there are more authoritative sources that a parent might consult, the ease with which we can find such information is indicative of the lack of stigma in grieving openly. Further, with the popularity of psychoanalysis and psychiatry also comes the formalization of the grieving process. This chapter revisits childhood mortality, with a focus on the modern developed world, and with a discussion of child death within the context of major world events: the Nazi Holocaust, school shootings, and war.

About 55,000 children die in the U.S. each year. According to the CDC's 2010 data set (the most recent data available), of the ten leading causes of death and injury, infants under the age of one die of congenital anomalies, pre-term birth, SIDS and injury, while the leading cause of death for children and adolescents ages one to eighteen is unintentional injury. Homicide and injury are among the top five causes for children ages one to eighteen. Suicide is the third leading cause of death for children and young adults ages ten to twenty-four. Other causes of death include heart disease, flu and pneumonia, and septicemia.[1]

Consolation and Grief

Chapter 9 discusses consolation literature: grieving manuals, poetry, and letters. Elisabeth Kübler-Ross, a medical doctor and psychiatrist, has written extensively on death and the grieving process, contributing many classic works to the genre of consolation literature. These works are written from both a medical (psychiatric) and humanitarian point of view. Kübler-Ross' *On Children and Death* is a manual not only for parents and siblings grieving a child's death, it is also provides information on how friends of the bereaved can help. The book also offers commentary on ways in which modern urban culture, particularly in the United States, does not facilitate the grieving process.[2]

One of the realities of a child's death from terminal illness that few people discuss is the high cost of dying—often between one hundred to two hundred thousand dollars, even with excellent insurance. Despite this financial burden, cash strapped parents will often overindulge a dying child, perhaps neglecting the emotional needs of his or her siblings. Kübler-Ross suggests that parents discuss the financial aspects of the illness with the children of the family by asking them to help find ways to save money. She also suggests that siblings help care for the sick child. When the child ultimately dies, siblings should, if they desire, be allowed to touch the body and bring gifts, notes, and perhaps a comfy pillow or beloved stuffed animal to inter with their brother or sister. Adolescents and children may want to help plan a funeral to some degree. It is not unheard of for classmates and considerate teachers to also join in the planning of a memorial.

When a child dies, whether unexpectedly or after a long illness, parents should be able to rock their child, hold them, kiss them, and sing to them. Even a stillborn baby should be given to the parents to hold, touch, and accept as a member of the family. One sensitive and knowledgeable funeral director's approach to removing a child's body from the home is to have the parents wash and dress the child, carry him or her to the car, and transport him or her (if possible) to the mortuary or funeral. When Kübler-Ross published her book in 1983, she noted that the process described above was followed by very few funeral directors. Now that so much more research is available to the profession, some funeral directors not only follow the above protocol, but offer other resources to help in grieving (such as bibliographies of books on mourning, prayers, and referrals to counseling services). Conversely, parents of children who have died during the commission of a crime must often identify their children in the sterile rooms in which bodies are laid out on a metal stretcher. The unnatural appearance of the child and the cold, formal environment is upsetting, painful, and impersonal.

Laura Smart notes that there are two contradictory views of grief: one view is that the bereaved must grieve in a particular way and that grief work should restore the bereaved to pre-bereavement state. The other view, generally accepted by the grieving and non-psychologists, is that grief should be over as soon as possible.[3] It is better to "move through the pain" than to avoid it by forgetting the death and its attendant rituals. It is essential to healthy grieving to acknowledge death, and having final moments with the deceased allows survivors (whether siblings, parents, or young friends) to mature and deal with other deaths. Making a shrine out of the child's room or having a "replacement" child before grieving has been processed is not conducive to a healthy life.[4]

Kübler-Ross, who has worked with the dying in most countries of the world, observes the change in culture in urban, and even suburban, communities in well-developed nations. Technology, prevalent transportation, and the move away from spirituality contribute to our inability to mourn in a healthy manner. Similarly, Suzuki notes the depersonalization of modern Japanese funerals, called McFunerals, which have become notable for their efficiency, depersonalization, and predictability, particularly with respect to mass-marketing of funeral services. In a McFuneral ceremonies last only one hour, and bodies are washed by professionals instead of loved ones. Mourners in some faiths or communities believe that the body of the deceased should not be left unattended. In McFunerals, however, in order to accommodate busy staff, it has been deemed acceptable for someone to just be "in the building". More recently, in response to these types of funerals new ceremonies have been established which are more personalized.[5]

In some parts of the world where children are abundant, there is always someone to care for them. In these regions children are seen as assets who will reciprocate that care for the elderly, eventually. Communities are no longer involved in birthing or welcoming children, nor are they involved when they die. Conversely, in well-established communities, where old customs are followed, in rural areas in particular, the community may help bury a child. Neighbors, and even children, might help dig the grave. A grandfather or other family member might build a coffin. By participating in the mortuary rituals, the community and family is permitted to grieve by doing something useful and meaningful. She notes that "death can be as simple and as uncomplicated as life is- if we don't make it a nightmare". Because of the fear of death, enabled by our present culture, parents who have lost a child might be reticent to have more children. Having children after the death of a child is a complicated reaction, discussed in depth in Chapter 8.[6]

Presently, there are support groups, such as "Compassionate Friends", to help parents grieve their children. For families and friends dealing with the particularly cruel aspects of losing a child who was murdered, there are support groups such as "Parents of Murdered Children". In these support groups, parents share stories of their children's lives, the circumstances of their deaths, and their own grieving. The stories from many parents include a discussion of clues their children left behind—many seemed to have a supernatural knowledge of their impending death (even if accidental). Notes, poems, drawings, and greeting cards appear to say goodbye, indicate knowledge of life beyond death—including visions of Jesus, white lights, and bucolic scenes. Parents lament not just the absence of the child but all that came with him; his friends, his mess and sarcasm. There are many "if onlies…" as parents wonder what they could have done to prevent death or to at least make their child's last days and months more loving.[7]

It is important when performing mortuary rituals that religious and cultural practice be respected, as funeral rites often have significant and symbolic meanings for the bereaved. For example, long ago the dead were buried under dirt and stone, the deeper the burial the more respected and feared the deceased. In a similar tradition, pebbles are placed on gravestones during Jewish funerals, presumably to weigh down the deceased.

Funerals are an opportunity to not grieve alone, and to share memories of the deceased. It is important to view the body, express emotions, and avoid sedatives—it will only delay grief. Mortuary rituals, particularly in the modern world, are not for the deceased; healthy expressions of grief are essential to the well-being of survivors. For divorced families, where the non-custodial parent may not be present at the death, he or she may also miss out on memory-sharing and a support network. Someone must make it their job to allow that parent to grieve by receiving the benefit of support and time with the body.[8]

As noted throughout the preceding chapters, funerals have always been costly. Kübler-Ross shares the conversations that she has had with poor, young girls who must bury a stillborn baby and want to know how to they will be able to pay for a funeral. While they might be directed to associations that will assist them, they are also reminded that "the body is cocoon". These girls are then relieved of their guilt of not being able to afford a real funeral.

Children's Funerals and Religious Beliefs

The spiritual beliefs of families, whatever they may be, often guide the bereaved through the grieving process. A researcher interviewing Australian families of recently deceased children investigated the role of children's funerals in grieving.

Some of the Roman Catholic funerals, once considered somber, were described as joyous occasions. In one case, an eighteen year old anticipating her death from leukemia selected her own music (disco), while at another funeral classmates of a seven-year-old boy sang a hymn. Funeral services for Roman Catholics differ from those that are Anglican in that the former say prayers for the soul of deceased. Greek Orthodox services include a vigil, and a traditional service without music, which are followed by additional services on the ninth and fortieth day.

Even though many religions call for specific rituals, parents and families attempt to personalize their goodbyes by dressing children to their tastes and offering goods, or personal possessions, to go with them on "their journey". Funerals for children have become more personalized, reflecting the music preferences and hobbies of the child. Families might recite poetry reflective of the life of the child. One eleven year old boy, aware that his death was impending, requested sparklers at his funeral so that "no one would be sad". After the burial, a witness noted, it was a spectacular sight to see all one hundred attendees light their sparklers.[9]

Jewish funerals, on the other hand, follow strict procedures. No music is permitted at the service. All family members must attend funeral services. An adult male, usually the father, recites the Kaddish, a mourner's prayer which must be read in the presence of at least nine other people, and must continue to be recited for a month after the death. A child is placed in a shroud with his prayer shawl around him. As in the practice of many other religions, the body must never be left unattended until the burial. Families sit shiva for seven days after the funeral, in which they remain home and perform no work. This mourning ritual allows the family time and space to grieve.[10]

With respect to infants who are miscarried, stillborn, or who do not live to thirty days, traditional Jewish response is that there is not to be any mourning as these children are not considered to have lived at all. The practice of not observing mourning rituals is based on tradition begun by rabbis during the Middle Ages, when many infants did not survive. Rabbis felt that relieving the parents of the obligation to mourn for a young infant, also relieved them from the burden of grief. Generally, in the Jewish faith, when neonates passed away, only three people attend the funeral. Traditional prayer is not recited, although tombstones have been found to sometimes mark the graves of these young infants. Modern Jews are attempting to change these practices. In keeping with modern research supporting the belief that parents must grieve their child's death, the Conservative movement has established new legal responses which carry the full authority of Jewish Law. These responses allow for the body to be buried according to standard practice, for the baby to be named, for Kaddish to be recited, and for the parents to sit shiva, if they wish.[11] For miscarried babies, or babies who were born prematurely, there is still some debate as to the appropriate mourning rituals, although some Jewish authorities state that families are encouraged to practice any rituals which would offer them consolation.

Funeral homes often offer services specific to memorializing children. While white caskets are traditionally used to bury children (symbolizing purity, as it always has), some funeral homes provide coffins decorated with teddy bears and other child-like themes. Some families might also choose to either audio or video record the service. As noted above, funeral homes can provide a wealth of information on bereavement, including recommended books, etiquette, and prayers appropriate for different family members. The website of one funeral home provides: "Prayer at the Grave of a Child", which states "I stand at the grave of my beloved child, I tenderly recall the joys he gave me during his lifetime…The passage of years will never fill the void in my heart."[12]

Treatment of Stillborn Infants

In Britain miscarried or stillborn infants, or those who die shortly after birth in the hospital, are often disposed of based upon the policy of the hospital. St. Mary's hospital, in Portsmouth, arranges the funerals for stillborn babies delivered in their maternity ward. Babies are buried six to a grave, sharing a communal headstone with a teddy bear carved into the corner which reads "In loving memory of our babies." All of the families' names are inscribed on the headstone along with the dates of birth/death. Parents tend to choose soft toys and miniatures, which are reminiscent of infancy, to decorate the graves of their children. While the gifts left on the graves indicate that the children are mourned, there is an aspect of ambiguity in the communal burial. To mitigate this ambiguity, some parents have begun to mark out a separate a space of the communal grave with a fence.[13]

Many women who have suffered miscarriages and stillbirths feel that their experiences are undervalued. It is only in the last forty years that women have been able to openly grieve the loss of child by miscarriage or stillbirth. Although friends and family may console the parents, the child is often forgotten soon after. Oftentimes well-meaning but misguided comments may indicate that the loss was a blessing (referring to the fact that a miscarriage is, at times, indicative of malformed or seriously ill fetus). Parent grief, however, is not easily resolved. Over time it may abate and be less acute, but it is always present. Women who choose to have an abortion grieve as well. Mental health professionals indicate that when a person is not afforded the opportunity to express grief to sympathetic listeners, resolution of the mourning is inhibited and often "shadows" the parent. It may even resurface at times when least expected. Symptoms of mourning reported by grieving mothers after stillbirth include, waking to the sound of a crying baby, continuing to feel the fetus kick even after it is born, and worrying if the baby is warm in its grave. Perhaps because the stillborn child is not given time to impress upon anyone other than the mother who carries him or her, mothers often perceive that others do not believe their grief is legitimate.[14]

Grieving Nurses Who Care for Dying Children

Healthcare providers that care for dying children, too, must move through the grieving process. Interviewing nurses in Scotland who provide terminally ill children with palliative care in the home, a private and culturally-centered space, Fiona Reid notes that these health care providers often mourn with emotion parallel to that of the parents. The grief of nurses who work with dying children might be compounded not only by the loss of the relationship with the family, as he or she will move on to another family to provide services, but by all of the previous deaths experienced during his or her career. The transition from healthcare environment to home care is so chaotic that often nurses provide the last twenty-four hours of end-of-life care on an informal and good will basis. In the cases of home care, nurses often become enculturated into the family's way of life and may find it difficult to remain neutral. Professional boundaries may become blurred as parents become reticent to receive medical advice, which might be in the best interest of the child but unpalatable (such as avoiding prolonging the life of a child in pain). Further, in their training, nurses are admonished not to cry, yet the anticipation of death of a child with whom they have bonded is difficult to navigate. Many nurses find a peer-network to be a productive outlet for their grief, although many try to avoid taking their "work" home with them. Only at the funeral do nurses feel that they may adequately express their grief. While nurses are directed to maintain professional boundaries and provide support at funerals, the ritual acts as a mechanism for closure. To manage their grief after the fact, nurses needed to draw upon their own considerable skills, often resolving their feelings alone, particularly when they feel a responsibility to help manage the grief of the families for whom they work.[15]

Of those children who contract cancer, between twenty-five and thirty-three percent ultimately die. Some of these children receive palliative care, which is more common for adults. To be eligible for palliative care often the patient must be considered terminal and in the last six month of life. Rarely do children's families seek out palliative care in these circumstances as they are often still attempting to cure the illness. Even when children do receive palliative care, the healthcare providers who work with them might often feel guilty for not having the skills to save the child, for "betraying" the trust of parents who left their loved one in the provider's care and, in their role as adults, for being unable to protect a child entrusted to them. This sense of failure, in addition to feelings of grief, helplessness, and guilt, can increase the anxiety and stress of the nurse. Some nurses might experience more grief when caring for dying children the same age as their own children. In order to avoid attachment, and therefore grief, a nurse might only attend to physical needs, avoiding the family.

As among nurses who provide homecare, these healthcare providers likely have the best knowledge about what pain management system works for the child and to what degree. They might know intuitively when it is time for the child to say his or her goodbyes. But often parents are resistant. They may try to continue to aggressively cure the illness, perhaps causing the child more discomfort. Despite these professional difficulties, which only facilitate personal stress and pain, nurses have the power to create a more comforting and compassionate environment for both the child and his or her parents.[16]

Euthanasia

The idea of relinquishing a child from life to avert excruciating pain is a difficult one for parents consider. For terminally ill children (and adults) palliative care only partially relieves pain. While near fatal doses of pain medication may be administered, children may suffer from dehydration and starvation, which may prolong life, possibly for weeks. At present, Belgium has become the first nation to legalize child euthanasia. Children under the age of eighteen, who are terminally ill and in intolerable pain, may advocate for their own deaths with the consent of their parents and doctor, provided they understand what euthanasia means.[17] Since 2005, the Netherlands has recognized the Groningen protocol, which allows a child under the age of one to be euthanized under a particular set of criteria. Eduard Verhagen, a physician and a lawyer, explains that ending the life of a terminally infant is not a difficult process and is rather peaceful. About ten to fifteen cases of euthanasia have been reported in the Netherlands each year from 1997 to 2004. Since then only two cases have been reported, although there has been an increase in late term abortions. Many euthanasia cases involve children with spina bifada, which has been detectable with prenatal tests offered for free in the Netherlands since 2007. Once the disorder is detected, expectant parents may choose to terminate the pregnancy. Some doctors and critics note, however, that hopeless cases of spina bifada are not detectable until an infant is born.[18]

Proponents of child euthanasia argue that a terminally ill child is often endowed with the maturity of an adult and may be able to make a decision about ending his or her own life with support from parents and physician. Critics, however, are concerned that emotionally, physically, and financially exhausted parents of an ill child might coerce a child to make this decision in lieu of palliative care. Opponents to the Groningen protocol also note that parents and physicians cannot reliably determine the suffering of a child subjectively.[19]

Euthanasia by the Nazis

The first systematic attempt to eliminate a specific population by the Nazi Regime was the selection and subsequent euthanization of between 5,000 and 8,000 disabled children. As part of the "racial hygiene" program, the Nazi's sought to cleanse genetic lines by removing children with both physical and intellectual disabilities. The infrastructure of the euthanasia program, while conceived of by Hitler and built by the Nazis, was supported and carried out by German physicians (Nearly forty-five percent of non-Jewish German doctors joined the Nazi party). Many of these physicians exploited the victims for the purposes of their own research, which included studies of twins and examinations of the brain before and after death. "Defective" newborns and children under the age of three were identified as potential "participants" in the program based on questionnaires filled out by midwives and doctors attending births. The state public health authorities then sent information about these children to the Reich Committee in Berlin, where staff with no medical training would select cases to be reviewed by experts. These experts would then select, unanimously, those children eligible for euthanasia. The children were then sent to one of twenty-two facilities. It was cruelly ironic that the stated purpose of these institutions was to save children from being permanently debilitated. Parental permission was required in order to transfer children to the euthanasia wards. Often permission was granted under false pretenses or threat. For example, parents might have been told that their children were to be treated for their disabilities. Children were killed via different methods including starvation, injection with medication (e.g., morphine, phenobarbital), and gassing. After the child died, a letter stating a fictitious cause of death would be sent to the parents. Children were cremated (after their bodies were used for research) and then parents would be billed for the cost of the "treatment".[20]

High Child Mortality in the Modern World: The Case of the Women of the Alto

Nancy Scheper-Hughes' rich work on the families of the Alto do Cruzeiro in Brazil demonstrates the disconnect between cultural expectations of expressions of mourning and experiences of grief in the face of high mortality. In the Alto do Cruzeiro, one of three shanty towns that surround the sugar plantation zone of Bom Jesus, mothers who have witnessed the deaths of many of their own young children, describe direct causes such as diarrhea and disease, and the more indirect causes such as poverty, malnutrition, a lack of money to purchase essential components for a baby's diet, and a lack of access to effective healthcare—in essence a lack of food. The mothers also acknowledge that their babies die of neglect when they must work and leave a sick or vulnerable infant alone. When asked about the death of their children, mothers often explained that their babies did not possess the proper "will to live"; the children lacked an internal force. They appeared weak and fussy, and lacked the will to nurse. These attributes work against the infants in many ways. The babies who appear to lack a life force are often preterm, low-birth weight, or dehydrated babies already at risk or in need of concerted care. On the other hand, these same qualities, which signal preterm, vulnerable babies, also cause mothers to withhold food and care, further hastening the child's demise. The food earmarked for the sick infant is instead given to stronger babies; the rich get richer and the poor get poorer, so to speak.[21]

Historically, and at present, the death of a child in much of Brazil was considered a blessing among all social classes, as its future well-being was promised. Deceased children, called *anjinho* (little cherub) were dressed in light blue or white shirts, with the cord of the Virgin around their bellies, covered with flowers and with a garland on their heads. They were positioned with their hands in prayer and eyes open. Parents wept joyfully, danced, drank, and played music. The celebration lasted several days. In rural Latin America some babies were handled like dolls, displayed on an altar, and even placed in a swing to signify the ascent to heaven. Mothers were expected to be joyful. These practices were found to be common in other Spanish speaking countries in both Latin America and Spain. It is possible that these beliefs were introduced by priests to console indigenous women in the face of high rates of child death after colonization. The practice of transforming a deceased child into an angel allowed mothers to idealize their children, making the journey to heaven tangible.[22]

In a marked contrast, in Bom Jesus, where bells used to ring frequently to signal the ascent of another *anjihho,* the chiming of the bells no longer sound. Infant burials are brief. The body is washed and dressed by a female child or the grandmother, and the funeral procession consists mostly of children. While previously the death of the child was met with joy and resignation, per Catholic teaching, in Bom Jesus the entire community, including the church and village bureaucracy, display indifference. The burial and grieving that subsequently follow the death of babies in the Alto is complicated. Mothers of the Alto are encouraged not to cry or grieve, lest their tears dampen the wings of the *anjelitos* (angels), obstructing them from flying on to heaven. The people of the Alto, especially the children, are at ease with the concept of death. Children commonly experience the death of a friend, young relative, or sibling; although in one case a child stated: "I don't want to lose another one".[23]

In Scheper-Hughes' interviews with these mothers she notes that their emotions toward their dead infants might be better described as pity instead of grief. These emotions have complicated origins not only in the incidence of high mortality and the repression of excessive demonstrations of grief, but in cultural expectations, and reconciliation with their domestic and socioeconomic environments. Some mothers state that they feel that they are freed from a burden when their baby dies. Their emotions are not delayed or displaced, and the women are not unfeeling. The psychological literature is rich with theories of grief, whether too much or too little, and its myriad expressions and attendant repercussions. Scheper-Hughes argues that women have traditionally been attributed the emotional tasks; loving their children and grieving their children. Therefore, society is uncomfortable when women do not grieve with the intensity of accepted norms. Many of the Alto mothers, however, explained that you might weep a little for an older child, but never for a young baby. Scheper-Hughes also explains a reconciliation the women make for their domestic situations. One husband "sadistically enjoyed" seeing his wife persistently pregnant; it seems that women of the Alto had little control over this function of their bodies. Scheper-Hughes suggests that the mother's refusal to grieve for her children is a way of stating "You can make me pregnant, but you cannot make me love all of them…or *keep* all of them either."[24]

Marilyn Nations refutes many of assertions and conclusions drawn by Scheper-Hughes in her study of dreaming as a vehicle for mourning in a culture where mothers are expected not to grieve openly for the children. She posits that the mothers (in her study of Ceara, Brazil) tolerate the death of their infants because they imbue it with "cultural significance". Resignation to death is a mostly Catholic belief (although examples are also seen in eighteenth century American Puritan and Quaker writings), and reactions to death are generally formed by cultural expectations. Analyzing the transcripts of interviews with forty-five women who had dreamed of their dead babies, Nations identified sixty-three themes including postmortem rituals (collecting keepsakes from each child, displaying photos of the deceased), maternal grief, and transfiguration of the dead child.[25] Nations also notes that for the Brazilian mothers she interviewed, death of a child is traumatic, as evidenced by the presence of all thirteen of BenEzers trauma signals, in the mother's narratives. These signals include: repetitive reporting of a particular traumatic event, inability to speak at all about the event, changes in voice during narration, intrusive images, and losing one's self in the retelling of the traumatic event.[26]

As these mothers are seemingly unable to prevent the high mortality of their children they must "rely on culture to relieve their suffering". Therefore, the mothers, in their dreams, transform their bruised, emaciated, and withered babies into chubby and cherubic, and often white, angels. Nations proposes that transfiguring dark-skinned sick babies into healthy white ones is a result of the inequitable social structure in Brazil, where the white skinned, blue eyed child is idolized, thereby eradicating the social stigma of indigenous status. Mothers have always dreamed of their deceased children as though still alive, although these mothers often recount how in dreams, the babies appear to be older than when they died. In this way babies continue to grow in the Afterlife. Nations also reported that once mothers received the highly anticipated first "visit" from their deceased child (about two to three months after the death), longing for their babies somewhat abated as they were able to confirm that their child continues on in the Afterlife.[27]

Additionally, if the child is unbaptized at death, it is believed that the child will wallow alone in purgatory for eternity. A mother has three chances to save her child's unbaptized soul: she can listen for its cry from the grave for the next seven years and baptize it on the seventh day, seventh month, or a year after its death. Mothers also note that breastfed babies must pass through purgatory in order to vomit the breast milk contaminated with their mother's sin. In some dreams symbols of funerals are eradicated in order "negate the irreversibility of death".[28] For example, candles are blown out; there is no corpse or casket, or evidence of the cause of death. Without these, there is no funeral and therefore no death. In this way hopelessness is alleviated because the mother does not feel that separation from her baby is absolute. In other dreams babies admonish their mothers for crying; tears weigh down the angel's wings and make them dirty, impeding them from getting to Heaven. Therefore, the mother acquiesces to the child's demand that they stop crying, not only in dreams but in waking-life, because it is the right thing to do. According to Nations, these dreams are a manifestation of grief, not otherwise realized. They save mothers from clinical depression, as most mothers are able to resign themselves to the death within a year after dreaming of the child, with less crying and with fond memories. "Only after the loss has been imbued with symbolic significance can the emotional pain be transcended and valued for the meaning it has been assigned."[29]

Day of the Dead in Mexico

The day of the dead, *dia de los muertos,* has been traced back to indigenous cultures, and may have its beginnings in an Aztec festival celebrating the "the Lady of the Dead" or *Catrina.* Celebrated on November 1st and 2nd, the days are also called All Saints' Day and All Souls' Day, respectively. In present day Mexico, November 1st is the day reserved for honoring infants and children. This day is called "Day of the Innocents" or "Day of the Little Angels". Celebratory practices include the creation of an altar for both children and adults. The children's altars include miniatures of items placed on the adults' altar, except for items like tobacco and adult foods. In Oaxaca, children's spirits arrive at 4 am on November 1st and leave at 8 am on November 2nd. One tiny candle is lit for each child. On the second day people decorate graves. Children receive the most elaborate decorations; tiny candles, *ollas* (food jars) and miniature gourds, and toys or figures representing the dead or the afterlife. Tiny pottery fruits and dishes are also set out on children's graves. "Feeding the dead" is an early Christian and early medieval practice. The Aztec ritual for the dead was practiced with the consideration that the afterlife is finite. For example, when a baby died the mother put a cane with her breast milk in it on the baby's chest for sustenance.[30]

Sandy Hook and School Shootings

On December 14, 2012 a disturbed young man entered Sandy Hook elementary school in Newtown Connecticut, an idyllic and seemingly safe community (with a crime rate a fraction of the national average), and gunned down twenty first graders and six teachers and administrators with a high capacity assault rifle. Soon after the shooting teachers and other school staff told how they hid young students in cabinets or in the bathrooms. One teacher, who had been murdered, had attempted to protect several children with her own body. The tragedy stunned the nation and refueled the right to bear arms/gun control debate. The rarity and extremity of Sandy Hook, the second deadliest school shooting in history, left the massacre without sufficient explanation.

When tragedy strikes, be it man-made or an act of god, the presence of the media and highly visible individuals such as the president is expected and observed. But in the case of Sandy Hook, along with the governor of Connecticut, the sheriff of Newton, the families of the victims, the president of the United States, and the journalists, the rest of the nation, and perhaps the world, effectively felt personally assaulted. An editor at a New York newspaper explained, the reason for our collective grief, horror, and indignation:

> Presidents don't cry. Journalists don't cry. Does anyone, nowadays, hear news of folks they've never met, and cry? Yeah, as it turns out, we do.…what makes the shooting…so different to me… [is that] they were not yet of the world, these kids. Their journey ended just a few feet from the start of the path, on what was supposed to be the safe stretch of trail.[31]

We adults are of this world, so too are the adolescents that are often plagued by self-destructive behavior. We are grieved, but we are not always surprised, when a shooting occurs at a high school or college or a public space where innocent bystanders are harmed. The murder of innocent children is another case entirely.[32] The closer in proximity, whether physically, psychologically, or personally we are to a tragedy (or stressful event) the more likely we are to suffer Post-Traumatic Stress Disorder (PTSD). In the case of the Newtown shooting, given the similarity of the community to many in which people in the U.S. currently live, or aspire to live, the presence of the president at the Sandy Hook Memorial, and the extensive media coverage (particularly with respect to social media, which put us in touch with the personal Facebook pages of the adult victims), the United States, and much of the world, suffered from PTSD.[33]

The tragic event has inspired many significant acts, whether artistic, charitable, or legislative. One moving example of the nation coming together to support the Newton community occurred during Christmas break, which quickly followed the shooting. The break allowed volunteers time to prepare a new place for Sandy Hook students to learn. During the holiday break more than one million paper snowflakes, from communities around the world, were sent to decorate the new school with a "blizzard of support". Each student and staff member was able to select snowflakes to take home with them in memory of this gesture. In 2013,

Patricia McLaughlin, an award-winning children's author, and Steven Kellogg, a children's book illustrator who previously lived in Sandy Hook, wrote a book for young children about Sandy Hook titled *Snowflakes Fall.* Written in metaphors, snowflakes symbolize both the tribute to the children and the children themselves.

Modern Conflict and War

As noted in Chapter 1, children born into or living during wartime are at high risk for death. During World War I, relatively few civilians (between five and nineteen percent of those killed) were killed by warfare. But since WWII that number has steadily risen about eighty percent. 7,736 children died during the blitz years in the United Kingdom. From 1980 to 1990 nearly 1.5 million children have been killed by wars, both declared and undeclared. The use of child soldiers has risen in the Middle East, in particular. During the Iran-Iraq war, 95,000 ten and eleven-year-old boy soldiers died.[34] Even in "peaceful" countries, such as the United States, children are at risk of violence at the hands of their parents or community. In 2011, 1,570 children died of abuse and neglect, and seventy percent of those children are under the age of four.[35] Children with a step-parent are more likely to die than those who live with one or both of their biological parents.

The most egregious example of conflict related mortality is the Holocaust in which of the six million Jews murdered at the hands of the Nazis 1.2 million were children. Many, many more children were brutalized, both physically and psychologically. Even as the Nazis were aware of their impending defeat in 1944 and were already retreating, "the Nazi machinery of death" in Hungary was inundated by the huge number of deportees waiting to be gassed in Poland. In order to expedite the process, Nazis threw living children onto burning fires. Children were the first targets of Hitler's "final solution", and as such their extermination has had a long lasting effect on the generations of Jews around the world.[36]

The book *I Never Saw another Butterfly* is a collection of poems and drawings by Jewish children who lived in the Terezin or Theresienstadt concentration camp. Terezin was actually presented as a model ghetto, with grass and flowers, in order to cover up the Nazi genocide. It was inhabited by scholars, writers, musicians and artists who were encouraged to be creative. The book is named for one of the poems written by a young inmate, Pavel Friedman, who wrote in 1942 "I never saw another butterfly...Butterflies don't live in here, in the ghetto..."[37] Butterflies are a symbol of eternal life.

As more children began to survive childhood, and as child death became rare and unexpected, grieving became an affliction that mental health professionals could help parents work through. Although more children have survived in the modern age, the circumstances that describe the deaths of modern children have become more complex and shocking. While genocide has been committed since the beginning of time, never has it occurred to the extent of the Nazi Holocaust. Further, the nature of gun culture and the weakness of mental health care have facilitated the advent of school shootings that have traumatized the world. It is not to say that the death of a child in the modern world is more distressing than it was in years past, but it is certainly less expected.

7

Indigenous Peoples of the World

Symbolism in Grief

From a modern Western perspective the mortuary practices of many indigenous groups around the world are among the most diverse. Indigenous peoples, as defined by the World Bank, are closely attached to ancestral territories and their natural resources, and are generally subsistence oriented. Indigenous peoples often are also the non-dominant groups in a society. Despite cultural evolution of surrounding groups, indigenous groups might eschew modern mortuary practices for their own traditional, mourning customs. The practices of indigenous peoples provide a window into the historic continuity of certain behaviors that precede colonialism or settlement by more dominant groups.[1]

Native North Americans

Religious beliefs play an essential role in mortuary behavior and mourning rituals for the great majority of the cultures discussed in this book. For peoples who have been the target of missionary expeditions, these behaviors and rituals can be confounded by traditional, indigenous beliefs and those of the adopted religions. In one example, Quincy Newell discusses how baptized Indians in California, between 1776 and 1821, approached major rituals accorded with birth, marriage, and death at Mission San Francisco. While over 600 Indians were baptized at the Mission, only some completely embraced the Catholic religion.

Few children lived past the age of two at the Mission. Disease in the crowded and unsanitary conditions, lack of dietary variety, and stress of acclimating to an unfamiliar culture were all cited as causes of the high mortality of both children and adults. Preferences for cremation or burial and other practices varied among Indians, but like the Apache (described below) mourning rituals of Indians at the Mission were elaborately violent affairs; belongings of the deceased were destroyed, mourners blackened their faces and cut their hair, although these practices were likely forbidden by the priests.[2]

Because they were considered too young to understand the sacraments, children did not receive penitence and extreme unction before death. Therefore, parents took their ill or dying children from the Mission to their native land. This practice indicated that in times of distress and death some Indians sought comfort with the familiar; their traditional cures for illness, customary mourning ceremonies, and burial in the land where they or their parents were born.[3]

Kiowa-Apaches have been noted to have extreme fear of ghosts. Accordingly, for them death was a traumatic experience. They believed that deceased ancestors came to escort them to the afterlife. Reaction to a death of a close relative was tempestuous; clothes were torn, naked bodies exposed, and perhaps even a finger was cut off. (Similarly, women in some aboriginal tribes will cut off fingers to represent those who died as a form of grieving). The ghosts of children, however, caused little concern "because of their innocence and lack of rancor". Consequently, children's deaths did not activate the same violent reaction as for those of adults. Despite the lack of fear of child ghosts, it was believed that children should be protected as they were vulnerable to a ghostly attack. Children were taught to look away from whirlwinds (thought to carry spirits), kept from funerals, and forbidden to touch a corpse. A newly mobile child's footprints were rubbed out, and if a child were left alone, a stick would be laid across his or her cradle.[4]

The burial practices of many tribes indicated concern for their young at death. For example, the Anasazi left many burial sites of infants. Infants were found wrapped in Yucca fibers and fur, and were buried carefully in their cradles where mourners left baskets, sandals and beads. Similarly, in the southwestern and southern United States, the Basketmakers (a group of hunters and gathers who lived in caves between 100–700 AD), often buried their infants (including fetuses) and young children in masses of soft fibers made from the leaves of Yucca plants or shrouded in fur, skin or feather-cloth blankets. These wrappings were used for both the living and the dead. Like the Anasazi, babies were left with grave goods. Generally the bodies were left in pits commonly used for storage, but some were left on the floor of a cave or placed in a crevice.[5] Other tribes, such as the Muskogean of the southeastern United States, buried their children in Pithoi (burial jars).

A desiccated three year old Pueblo child was found on an elaborate cradleboard with a cotton wood-bark sunshade placed on his head and adorned with a bracelet around the wrist. This burial was considered unusual, as other burials of the time were less extravagant and did not have grave coverings. Archaeologists infer that the child may have been disabled, perhaps unable to walk, because of the placement of the toddler on a cradleboard.[6] Usually only infants were buried on a cradleboard or in a grass nest, while others were placed in twined bags or, more often, in an animal fur shroud.

Babies of many native peoples were often believed to be reincarnations of ancestors. Therefore, these children were never hit, or else it was thought that the soul of an offended ancestor would depart the body and leave behind a dead child. In another example, Huron and Meskwaki mothers buried dead infants beside footpaths in the belief that the spirit would be reincarnated by entering the body of a woman passing.[7] These beliefs also were evident in naming practices (discussed further in Chapter 8).

Tribes of Africa

For the Vezo of Madagascar "boneless" babies (newborns) were not considered human until they got older. Until then, they were strongly tied to their mothers. As a non-human, if a baby died before the age of one, it could not be buried within the family tomb. For some cultures, superstition surrounded the remains of children. Up until the 1920s, the Yoruba of Nigeria would leave a dead baby in a bush because a burial would offend earth shrines that ward off death and bring fertility. Presently, the Yoruba bury their dead infants in backyards or in the forest, but it is still done unceremoniously, without ritual bathing, shaving of the head or the dressing that usually would accompany a funeral. In many parts of western Africa, in fact, no infant may be buried below ground for fear of upsetting fertility-inducing Earth shrines. The Lodagaa of Ghana bury young infants, who have not yet been weaned, at a crossroads beneath a pile of dirt, their cradles anchored above them with stakes to prevent the babies from returning. These children are called by the Yorubas *abiku* "born to die". They are believed to be demons, born over and over again into the wombs of particularly cursed mothers. Babies of these mothers are protected with charms and given names such as "one who comes and goes". Feasts are held for these children in order to appease the *abiku* spirits.[8]

Like some prehistoric Neolithic groups and peoples from Oceania (described below), many tribes from Africa buried children within the house or in places to facilitate rebirth into a new child. The Bogushu of Uganda, for example, tended the graves of dead children until the soul was born into a new sibling. Since it was then believed that the buried child no longer possessed a soul, their bones were dug up and discarded. Similarly, in Congo the souls of dead infants were believed to be reborn into each new sibling within a family. Some West African tribes hid the remains of dead infants in bushes along a path to allow souls to leap into passing women.[9]

Infanticide among Indigenous Groups

South America

There are about 240 ethnic groups in Brazil. Accordingly, there is a diversity of indigenous groups which, despite colonization 500 years ago, have minimal contact with other groups or the Brazilian society in general. The practice of infanticide, extremely prevalent among these groups, has been widely questioned by legal authorities. Saulo Feitosa and colleagues describe a seminar in 2005 on legal pluralism during which an attorney working in Brazil asked a representative of the International Labor Organization (ILO) how to approach cases of infanticide among indigenous groups. The ILO representative responded that human rights should be respected and infanticide should be addressed, however, an anthropologist in attendance disagreed and argued that indigenous mothers have "full autonomy" on deciding whether their children should live.

Mothers of the Yanomami, for example, give birth in the forest. If the mother does not "welcome the child into her arms", it is as though the child were never born. The anthropologist explained that children permitted to survive are given a second "birth" by being accepted into the community. Rejection by the mother after birth precludes the community's acceptance. In a sense, the life of a child is a cultural "construction". There are rarely records of mothers being prosecuted for infanticide as the act is seen as a communal decision.[10]

Girls born to single Zuruhua mothers, another Brazilian indigenous group, are almost always marked for death because their lives are considered too difficult, both for themselves and for the community. When a female is born to a single mother, she is left still attached to the placenta in a thicket until either the mother or a relative kills her. The societal and cultural expectation of this practice indicates that an absent father precludes a daughter from being accepted into society. A boy with no father, however, is allowed to live, although he is given a lower status. He is saved because of the perception of male usefulness. In the one case of a Zuruhua widow who chose to raise her two daughters, both girls committed suicide as adults. Because this group has a long history of high rates of suicide, children learn the concept very early and often role play their own deaths and funerals. The community's relationship with suicide stems from a massacre that took place over one hundred years ago.[11]

While it is widely known that females are more likely than males to be victims of infanticide, among the Waiwai, the fifth child of a family is sacrificed if he or she is the same gender as the older four siblings, regardless of sex. Because breastfeeding for about two years is common, subsequent pregnancies are postponed. If a child is conceived during this period, a mother might choose to kill it. In these indigenous populations, infants are killed when the mother is unwilling or unable to care for the child, or when the baby would be unable to survive in the environment into which he or she was born (whether because of a birth defect or a deceased mother).[12]

The Guanas in South America reportedly buried most of the female children alive when birth rates needed to be controlled. In this society families may have up to four children, one of them at the whim of the mother; however, the decision to have three more is up to the father.[13] For the Ayoreo, a tribe in Bolivia and Paraguay, the mothers and female kin chose the circumstances over which they would perform infanticide. The women never reported on their own acts, though, as it would "make them sad".[14]

Conversely, when beloved babies died, the Laymi, an Amerindian people of northern Bolivia, buried deceased children (called *anjelito* or little angels) with white paper wings attached to their shrouds so they could fly to heaven.[15] This practice also was common among many groups in Brazil. As discussed in Chapter 6, it was thought that a child's death was a cause for joy and celebration. Consequently, mothers were discouraged from grieving openly.

Oceania

The Kaliai of Western New Britain had no ritual burial for infants. The boundary between infants and full humanity was identified by the ability of a person to discuss his or her dreams. Therefore, there was a lack of consequences for infanticide.

Infanticide was usually practiced when "unnatural" births occurred; multiple births or children born with deformities.[16]

The Papuans of British New Guinea are reported to have buried their children alive when a parent or other caregiver passed away so that he or she could care for the parent in the afterlife. Additionally, the Papuans practice cannibalism. Murder is deemed as a mode of releasing feelings of anger, grief or anxiety.[17]

Among the Pacific Atoll islanders abandonment was rare, although when practiced, infanticide was rooted in superstition. For example, as in many other indigenous cultures, if twins or a deformed infant was born, the newborn(s) were killed. The Maori and Polynesians practiced foundation sacrifices, offering a son when a building was constructed. The Tokelaes of Lind Islands controlled their population by limiting the number of children born to a family to four. After that number was reached, infants were buried directly after birth. The Tonga strangled sick babies. If the Tonga perceived an angry god was present, a two year old was sacrificed by strangulation. In Papua New Guinea infanticide of girls was practiced until recently.[18]

While the wartime killing of infants by outsiders was and is common, some groups in distress, such as the Tlingit of North America and the Maori, have killed their own crying infants to avoid being found out when hiding. In another example, any infants and children who slowed down the Tasmanian's escape from Europeans were killed.[19]

In the mythology of the Aborigines of Australia and Groote Eylandt the ancient earth mother gives birth to all of the spirit babies. The Aborigines believe that the spirit of a victim of infanticide goes to the "store of spirit children" that are waiting to be reborn. A recurring theme of the burial of the young, especially among those who are victims of infanticide or sacrifice, is that the young are released to negotiate between the living and the dead.[20]

North American Indians

Some Apache mothers seemed to demonstrate a contradictory dynamic with their children. Anthropologists have observed that while Apache mothers nursed their children frequently, and were very close, physically, with their infants, many mothers guiltlessly abandoned or gave away children. In fact, many mothers stated that they had "forgotten" that they ever had the children they had given away. This has been explained as the Apache mother's belief that children only require physical care, but not emotional relationships or attachment with their children. As discussed in Chapter 6, like the women of the Alto in Brazil, grief and relationships with infants, where child mortality is high is complicated and not easily explained.[21]

As among peoples in other regions of the world, births which differed from the norm perpetuated distress among Indian communities. For example, the Shoshone of the Great Basin rejected twins or deformed infants and buried them in badger holes. Additionally, Apache girls were instructed on how to end the life of a twin or abnormal or ill child. Those infants who were born normal and kept by their mothers were carefully cared for (as noted above). Those who died were wrapped onto their cradleboards and hung upon a tree.[22] The Creek and Muskogee tribes were matrilineal societies; as such, mothers were permitted to commit infanticide before the child reached the age of one.

Like the ancient South and Central American peoples, child sacrifice was performed to appease gods or royalty. In Florida, the Timucua natives sacrificed their first born children to the chief. The infant was placed on wooden stumps and slain in the presence of the king while women danced and the mother wept. The Natchez commoners sometimes offered one of their children for sacrifice to accompany dead royalty to their graves.

While children born out of wedlock or beget from infidelity were generally targets for abandonment, Eskimo babies of any paternity were accepted, and any person who abandoned such a child to the cold was quickly punished.[23] Apparently this rule applied only to male babies, however, as female infanticide appeared to be quite common. Eskimos, and other groups who relied on hunting, were constantly in danger of losing too many males. Due to the high rate of male death, female infanticide was practiced to even out the distribution of the sexes.[24] This tended to cause a shortage in females, though, as evidenced by the theft of wives from other tribes by young Eskimo men.

Tribes of Africa

Infanticide in Africa was less often practiced than on other continents, but as with other groups, unusual births were met with concern by some tribes. When twins were born, the Zulu, Sotho and Pedi killed one twin. Like the Shoshone of the Great Basin, the Vendu and Lobedu killed both twins as the mere occurrence of multiple births was considered abnormal. The Xhosa, Bomuana, Thembu, and Mfangu considered all babies a blessing; however, two euphorbia trees were planted when twins were born. If one of those trees died, the corresponding twin was killed. For the !Kung unwanted children were buried immediately after birth.[25]

To control population, select genders, and to space children African hunter-gathers (Bushmen), pastoralists (the Chagga and Malagasy of Madacascar), and the South African Bamba performed infanticide. Because a large family was and is essential for agricultural groups, most agriculturalists and pastoralists do not practice infanticide. Furthermore, due to colonialism and the loss of man power to slavery and new diseases, some groups could not afford to commit infanticide. Infant mortality among agriculturalists and pastoralists ranged from twenty-six to fifty percent.

Burial Places

As in prehistoric times, there are many examples of indigenous children buried in areas, particularly in the home, meant to facilitate rebirth of the dead. Keisan children of Indonesia are buried under their parents' sleeping spaces, while the Aaru hang dead infants above the sleeping area. The placement of deceased offspring was intended to both protect surviving children and to induce fertility in the parents; perhaps allowing the soul to enter the new child's body.[26] Melanesians hung up favored deceased children in their homes either in a canoe or enclosed in the figure of a swordfish. Similar practices are also found among the indigenous Maori and the Sacastrans of the Balkans, where deceased infants are placed in bags and hung above their parent's bed to dry for forty days. Some Indonesian societies, such as the Timorese, bury the placenta and umbilicus in symbolic areas of, or near, the house in order to protect the newborn.[27] (As noted in earlier chapters, the ancient Roman practice of burying infants under the walls of the house, and the Russian peasant practice of burying stillborn children under the floor served the same purpose). For similar reasons, the indigenous tribes of Australia place the bodies of children in "wooden troughs and then deposited [them] on platforms of boughs arranged in the branches of trees."[28]

Among the Rotinese in Eastern Indonesia, child spirits were often deemed spiteful and a danger to mothers and their future children. A child who had died before three months of age was buried under a ladder of the house, while a child who died between the ages of three months to one year was wrapped in cotton and buried next to a cotton plant.[29] In Java, children who died unnamed were buried behind the family hut. In the Andaman Islands children were buried beneath the hearth in the belief that the soul would enter the mother's body, while she cooked, and would be reborn. The children of Vanuatu and Kois of Southern

India, were buried at the threshold of the house to be reincarnated within another woman's womb.[30]

Funerary practices in Melanesia and Australia are widely disparate. In some areas preserved bodies have indicated behaviors reflective of cultural values associated with death: in some societies mummification has been ascribed to those of higher social status, while in other tribes or cultures it has been commonly practiced among people of any status. Mummification has also been practiced to avoid haunting by spirits. In one example of child mummification, an aboriginal Australian infant was found preserved lying on a net bag filled with long grasses, placed on its side covered by another layer of grasses and a wallaby hide.[31]

Little is written of the grief of indigenous mothers. This is perhaps because infants may not be considered humans in some societies until they reach certain milestones: the age of one, the ability to speak or walk, or have the ability to recollect and report dreams. This is further confirmed by the acceptance of infanticide in many societies, especially for children under the age of one. The Shona of Zimbabwe, for example, practice Christianity but also hold fast to traditional beliefs. Despite the cause of death, whether natural or superstitious, the mother often is blamed is inhibited from grieving openly for a very young child.[32] Dreamworks, the exploration of the emotions that dreams evoke, has importance in the process of healing for indigenous mothers, particularly among Native North Americans and aboriginals in Malaysia, Australia, and Indonesia where spiritual beliefs are based on mystical surrealism.[33]

Part II

Indicators of Parental Attitudes toward Child Death

8

Indicators of Parental Concern

Naming and Replacement

In October 2011, 220 Indian girls chose new names after shedding given names that meant "unwanted" in Hindi. Names like "Nakusa" blight the self-worth of many young girls in India named by parents or grandparents disappointed by the birth of a daughter. Names, so integral to one's identity, is a confirmation of one's existence as well as an indicator of parents' expectations. The value Indian parents place on girls is not only reflected in the names given to their daughters, but in the gender ratio; there are 914 girls for every 1,000 boys. This disparity is due to selective infanticide and abandonment.[1]

Naming in Different Cultures and Time Periods

Naming practices differ among various cultures and across time periods. At times, naming may reflect the state of childhood survival in a region. In the case of Indian girls, the naming of infants and children might reflect the values of the culture with respect to the importance of gender or lineage (e.g., the denial of a family name to a child born outside the bounds of marriage). Use of biblical names, or adaptations of male names for females (e.g., changing Samuel to Samantha), and names used to reflect expectations of positive personal attributes such as courage or intelligence are also indicators of cultural ideals. In some societies children are named after grandparents because it is believed that associating a name with a soul facilitates the reincarnation of that ancestor. Child naming practices are not random, "but instead conform to deeper cultural rules".[2] Parents in societies with high infant mortality may often delay the naming of a child until the threat of injuries or illness has passed. It is the fear of death that is often so acutely reflected in the name of a child, as illustrated in the following examples.

Like the many other societies discussed below, ancient Romans did not give an infant a name until the seventh or eighth day of life, due to the high mortality rate of newly born infants. Parents who allowed their children to die unbaptized were subject to punishment by the church. However, the penance was less severe if an infant died before the seven day period.[3] As noted in Chapter 4, baptism of the newly born could often be problematic in medieval Europe. Names in the baptismal record of a town were often the only evidence of a person's existence and records were often unreliable. If children were not baptized before death, it was unlikely that there would be a record of their existence.

It is a common perception that there was indifference toward medieval children based upon naming practices. For example, the custom of giving a newborn the name of a deceased sibling was a tradition meant, perhaps, to give life to an otherwise "abandoned" name, particularly when many children from the same family died with the same name.[4] Medieval parents often followed the pattern of doubling up on names for two or more children. Unlike the Massachusetts Puritans (described below), however, they distinguished one from the other by use of the terms "major" and "minor". Thus, naming may also reflect the practice of replacement (discussed below).[5] Other naming practices include evoking the memory of an ancestor or hero, or conveying good wishes such as "may God guard you".[6]

In early colonial America (and Europe) some children were not named until they reached the age of one. If an infant died before this milestone, his headstone would simply state "Our Baby".[7] There was also a strong tendency to use religious names such as Faith, Charity, Hope, or those from the Bible. Like medieval families, it was not uncommon for colonial American parents to name their children after deceased siblings. For example, from 1720 to 1800 seventy-five to eighty-five percent of children were named for a deceased sibling.[8] This included girls' names that were transformed from their deceased brothers' (e.g., Christian/Christine, Frank/Frances). The reasons for this repetition are diverse. First, parents recognized the high likelihood of a child's death and wanted to guarantee that they would have a same-name successor. In the eighteenth century nearly ninety percent of dying children named for a parent, had their names also bestowed to a sibling. "As death became romanticized in the late 18th and 19th centuries, the deadness of deceased children did not seem so complete. Parents before 1800 may have appreciated the uniqueness of the living child. But since death was so absolute, they found it appropriate to give a succeeding child the name of his or her deceased sibling".[9] As attitudes towards death changed, so too did naming practices.

There were no differences in repetitive naming practices between infants (who had a higher mortality rate) and children between one and five; "thereafter, age at death actually increased the likelihood of necronymic successor, especially for children not named after parents. This pattern is the opposite of what we would expect to find if the modern sense of uniqueness had obtained".[10] One might assume that the personality of an infant would be less apparent to a mother and father, than that of an older child. He or she would not yet have adopted the identity that comes with the name.

Puritans began a tradition of using uncommon names that reflected their view of children. Names such as Thankful, Chastity, and Tribulation Wholesome indicated Puritan parents' gratitude for their children. While Puritans had a reputation of being harsh with children, they also demonstrated parenting that elevated them among their contemporaries.

Native American families from Eskimo, Chukchi, and Koryak tribes, among others, named their children for deceased family members, since babies were believed to be ancestral reincarnations. These children were never hit as it was believed that the soul of an offended ancestor would depart the body, leaving behind the dead child. Since infant and child mortality was high among all native children, they were often called "baby" or "little one" until the age of five or as late as ten. Similarly, the Inca left their children unnamed until they were two or three years old, when they were weaned. A temporary name was given to Incan children until a permanent one was bestowed at puberty.[11] These practices demonstrated a deep affection for family in general, a reverence for ancestors, but also a cognizance that their infants may be on borrowed time.

Infanticide among some indigenous peoples in Brazil is often seen as a communal decision to not accept the child (as discussed in Chapter 7). In cases where children were "eligible" for infanticide (for reasons of being born with a deformity or without a father) but permitted to live, those children were not named until the age of two. Among the Katukina people, withholding a name is a way of socially "killing" a child; it marks the child as unwanted. Since infanticide is no longer practiced among the Katukina, "failure to give a name is an indirect way of exposing the child to death." Accordingly, for other indigenous groups in Brazil, giving a name right away suspends the possibility for infanticide.[12]

In China, belief that "treasured" children are desired by the devil enlists parents to engage in a ruse of renaming children to suggest indifference. Infants may be named "Dog" or "Pig" to falsely signal disgust for a child. Boys may have been dressed as girls, or parents might go through a show of a sham adoption, all in order to feign a lack of interest or disdain so that the devil would reject the child.[13] As in modern India, in modern China the desire for the birth of a baby boy is reflected in the names of baby girls. Presently, there are more than six million women in China named *Lai Di* or *Jao Di*, which means "Boys come, come, come".[14]

In early twentieth century Japan, baby girls remained unnamed for thirteen days and boys for thirty-one. The death of a child is perceived as an omen from an angry Heaven and presents a threat to the next child to be born. Parents mitigated that threat by feigning abandonment to a bamboo grave where a friend of relative could "stumble" upon it and claim it. The child would then be presented to the parents as a replacement for the lost chlid. These same infants were than given co-names to indicate their status, such as *sute* (abandoned), *sutejiro* (abandoned second-born).[15]

Colonial Uganda and the Zulu of South Africa

Children in many African societies have meaningful names that generally point to circumstances or people relevant at the time of birth, which is opposite of the Western practice of naming as function of labeling. Shane Doyle's study of parental attitudes toward child death in colonial Uganda, however, demonstrates the expectation of death. Examining the baptismal records of the Bunyoro society in Western Uganda, Doyle found that nearly one-third of names given during the colonial period referred to death.[16]

Names given to children such as *Kembandwa* and *Mugasa* indicated that the birth was a result of prayers to traditional spirits. As in China and Japan, where babies were named after rats, dogs, monkeys, or other unpleasant objects, many Bunyoro parents gave their children names to deter death by feigning contempt. Consequently, *Kunobere* (I hate this child) was a common name. Some names referred to the deaths of siblings such as *Nyamayarwo* (children are meat for it [death]) or *Nkafiika* (I am the only survivor). Over ten percent of names given signified a belief that the child would die: *Ndoleriire* (I am waiting to see what happens), *Bagada* (what a waste of energy), or *Byeitaka* (this child belongs to the soil). Interestingly, these types of names, which pointed to the parent's surety that the child would die, were more common in 1920–1934, the time period following the years of the highest mortality.[17] Doyle explains that the predominance of death-names in the baptismal registry may have been a self-fulfilling prophesy to some degree. Children who were more likely to die would have been baptized much earlier than other children. Doyle observed, however, that parents of babies whose names indicated an expectation of death waited thirty-one days longer than the average family to baptize.

The decline of death-names revealed that a new "sense of privacy, part of a self-conscious modernity, was valued: 'Such [death] names were given in the past because people had the spirit of saying let me expose to the whole world what is going on here. Today people want to cover [it] up.'"[18] It is possible that Ugandans' conversion to Christianity changed the naming practices as well. In modern times, positive names, such as *Asiimwe* (thanks be to God), have become common. Bereaved parents are now encouraged to see death as a positive, temporary parting to heaven. In the past Ugandan parents did not know the cause of their child's death, so naming indicated a call to the spirits. With the rise in AIDS cases diagnosed, and the subsequent HIV awareness education, parents came to understand that death was not mysterious; it had a cause (be it AIDS or another illness). Bunyoro's example exhibits a rapid change in societal perceptions of death. After 1940 the use of death names declined, signifying a rise in infant survival rates. The use of death names, however, did not re-emerge during the AIDS pandemic, when infant mortality rates again increased. Doyle argues that along with a belief in the afterlife, this society experienced an evolution of perception about death. Bunyoro parents were aware that they had suffered much higher mortality rates and low fertility in the past.[19]

In Zulu, a Bantu language of South Africa, some examples of symbolic children's names are translated as: "Where does he come from?", which questions the legitimacy of the child; "Nail" (the mother was part of a polygamous marriage and had 'hit the nail on the head' by having a boy); and "Grow up" (the mother had told her father and brother that they must grow up because they were now grandfather and uncle).[20] The name "Awaited" was given to a child whose parents had waited a long time for a living child. It appears that in the Zulu culture, like in colonial Uganda, the child's name reflected the circumstances of birth, personality traits, perhaps hopes for the future and even strained family relationships. Like the Japanese, Chinese, and Ugandans, the Zulu also named children with the intent of warding off evil spirits. Names meaning "vile" or "excrement" were common, as was presenting a girl's name to a boy. Because infant mortality was relatively lower for the Zulu than for other African cultures, names tended to emphasize the positive.

Replacement

It is well known among demographic researchers that a rise in mortality often precipitates a rise in fertility. Replacement strategy is a term used to define the act of purposefully replacing a child who has died. It is a natural biological and emotional response. In some cases the strategy has been used as insurance in anticipation of child deaths. Parents might "hoard" children, particularly in societies with high mortality. Conversely, in families where multiple child deaths have occurred, a family might employ birth control methods in order to avoid the risk of the emotional toll of further losses.[21] Sometimes the replacement effect is caused by a shortened breastfeeding period as a result of infant death, which in turn causes fertility to return postpartum. This phenomenon has been observed universally, particularly after major traumatic world events, such as the Holocaust and World War II.

Knodel, a sociologist at the Population Studies Center in Michigan, explains that the replacement effect is a fertility response, voluntary or involuntary, while replacement strategy is the deliberate conception of a child to replace one who had died. In terms of pure numbers Knodel acknowledges that replacement is rarely complete as children might die after parents are biologically incapable of procreating. When parents employ the method of having extra children as a means of insurance, they run the risk, demographically speaking, of having fewer children than they desire (or than what is needed to support the community, as observed in the Middle Ages during and after the plague). Population strategists argue that replacement strategy is a more reliable means of ensuring that the desired size of the family remains stable. Further, some demographic researchers argue that there are cultural differences between fertility strategies. During periods of economic or marital distress, fertility is often delayed. Therefore, replacement strategies are not always a reliable indicator of demographic trends.[22]

HIV and Replacement in Zimbabwe

A study examining parents in Zimbabwe, where twenty-five percent of adults were HIV positive in the twenty-first century, revealed that parents who experienced the death of a child were reluctant to have another lest it too succumb. In

Zimbabwe childbearing is an important part of life, and children are considered essential to the relationships between mothers and fathers. Despite parent education and abstention from childbearing, the rate of mother-child HIV transmission has not decreased. Parents, however, stated that they would have fewer children given the rising mortality rates due to AIDS. Because both children and adults die as a result of AIDS, the replacement and insurance strategies are not viable methods of increasing or maintaining the size of families, particularly when a parent dies and there are fewer resources to care for surviving children. Instead many parents choose to focus on their living children and their own health. About thirty percent of children born to HIV positive mothers also contract HIV. Due to misunderstandings about the fatality of the virus and its transmission, when HIV positive parents have children who do not contract HIV, they mistakenly believe that they too are virus free and continue to have more children. The dynamic surrounding HIV's unique effects, and lack of knowledge of how it is contracted, as well as the typical fertility responses to child mortality, confound reproductive decision making for Zimbabwean parents.[23]

The Replacement Child

The psychological impact on a replacement child can be significant, whether children are expressly sired to replace a deceased child or given the designation because they are the youngest sibling. While rare in the psychiatric literature, some researchers note that the practice of replacing deceased children in the modern developed world is likely more common than is reported. Replacement children are often raised by fearful and overprotective parents in a home where photographs of the deceased sibling loom over survivors. Psychologists argue that these children may not develop their own identities as they are expected to emulate those of the departed brother or sister. Mental health professionals also acknowledge an "anniversary reaction". When the anniversary related to the deceased child (whether the birth or death of the child) or the traumatic event occurs, there is an emotional reaction. An anniversary reaction does not always occur in the cases where there are replacement children. Indeed the two phenomena are mutually exclusive; however, a parent's anniversary reaction may impute an intense role for the child to play in the family.[24]

Elva Poznanski provides the example of a family who lost their five year old child, who apparently foretold her impending death in a car accident. In the same accident her twin suffered traumatic brain damage. After the accident the family had another child whom they considered naming after the deceased sibling, but instead named her "Susie". The family often realized self-fulfilling prophesies in which the father would predict some type of trouble that would then occur (usually related to his young daughter). Each year on the anniversary of the accident, the family would not drive anywhere, the day would be fraught with sadness and depression, and often the father would call Susie by the name of his deceased daughter. The living daughter later engaged in destructive behaviors and dangerous relationships, and was institutionalized for a period of time, presumably as a result of her role as the replacement child. Conversely, Poznanski also describes how another mother began to demonstrate signs that her youngest child (born after the death of another child) was a "replacement". Her pediatrician intervened and discussed with her the dangers of projecting her deceased daughter's personhood onto her younger daughter. Cognizance of what this mother might be doing to her child likely prevented some of the psychological trauma that Susie experienced as a replacement child.

Susie's parents never fully grieved; they merely imbued their deceased daughter's memory on her, and with it, their expectations. Given that the deceased child is generally idealized by the parent, these expectations are almost impossible to meet. Further, Susie's destructive behaviors, and relationship with a boy who threatened to kill her, made it a realistic possibility that she might die, as replacement children may also internalize their parents' fears. Because of this unhealthy cycle of behaviors, parents cannot raise a new child without the possibility of he or she becoming a replacement child (with all the attendant issues), until they have acknowledged the loss of the dead child, suffer a period of bereavement, and then fully engage in other healthy relationships.[25]

9

Consolation Literature

Sympathy Letters, Poetry, and Books on Parental Grief

Consolation literature has taken on various forms throughout history. It may be seen in letters between or to grieving parents, lamentation poetry, books of advice on how to deal with the death of a child, or even how to grieve appropriately in public. Some historians consider consolation literature a form of psychotherapy; an avenue by which parents may grieve. For example, Yiddish Holocaust lullabies appear to have been written to sustain morale, "support the psychological structure, and integrate the traumatic loss of a people threatened with psychic disorganization during the Holocaust".[1] This chapter discusses selections of consolation letters, manuals, and poetry written to, about, and by grieving parents.

Plutarch's Consolation Letter to His Wife

One of the most well-known examples of consolation literature was written by Plutarch, the Greek historian, philosopher and politician, who eventually became a citizen of Rome. Upon hearing of his two year old daughter's death, for which he was absent, he wrote a letter to comfort his wife. This letter has been published, commented upon, analyzed and criticized through various perspectives. One interpretation of the letter is that it may be seen as a public show of steadfastness and dignity; a commentary upon grieving. Another more obvious interpretation is that the letter is a moving attempt to console his grieving wife.

Because Plutarch was away during the death, burial, and subsequent period of mourning, the letter is the only method by which he could hope to console and support his wife. At the same time, as a public figure, he knew that his letter may be open to public consumption. With this knowledge he writes reminders to his wife that she was not prone to "extravagance or superstition, for which I know you have no inclination", indicating his expectation that she would behave appropriately. On several occasions in the letter he remarks on her ability to demonstrate "right female behavior", while acknowledging the sadness he feels over the loss of the child, as well as the great loss his wife must feel. These suggestions seem to be a call to other mothers to not employ "wailing women", for example, in a time of death. He also mentions his wife's care of the child and their other children (noting that she breastfed their children, which was uncommon among the aristocracy in ancient Greece). He calls upon his wife to be an example for other grieving mothers, as "grieving does not help" and "moderation of emotion may help deal with it". Plutarch's descriptions of some memories of the child also add value to the letter as a memento that may be read over and over again by his wife.[2]

The perception of ancient Greek and Roman parents as unemotional in response to the deaths of their children is common. Yet, as Baltussen asserts, Plutarch's letter demonstrates otherwise. "Although it is difficult to gauge the level and sincerity of such emotional investment, it would be [remiss]...to deny the parents of classical antiquity any feelings for their young children", given Plutarch's loving and descriptive commemoration of his child.[3] Plutarch's consolation, however, is tempered by this statement: "extravagance of distress...will be more grievous to me than what has happened", as Roman parents were forbidden to formally mourn a child less than three years of age.[4]

Plutarch's consolation letter expands upon the writings of Crantor and Cicero. Crantor, a Greek philosopher from Soli, Cilicia, wrote what is considered his most famous work "On Grief" to his friend Hippocoles', as a consolation upon his son's death.[5] Crantor expounded that grief was natural and that "the absence of pain comes at a high price; it means being numb in body, and in mind scarcely human."[6] Around the time of his daughter's death in 45 BC, Cicero, who borrowed heavily from Crantor, wrote of sorrow as a disease within the mind, in need of treatment.

Upper class ancient Romans had the benefit of non-public outlets for their grief, such as consolation literature and funerary rituals. On occasion, the wealthy grieved openly without self-control. Upon witnessing a display of mourning the

Roman philosopher Seneca wrote a letter to his friend on the futility of grieving at the death of an infant. Seneca argued that the child was so young that "no hopes could have been invested in him; he might have turned out badly as sons often did." He goes on to acknowledge that while it is natural to show grief, one should not do so excessively. Further, a bereaved parent should remember the dead and reflect on his life. Thus, while it is clear that the father was distraught over the death of his young son, even Seneca, appealing to his rationality, admits to the sad nature of death.[7]

Consolation Manuals for Parents

Between the thirteenth and sixteenth centuries more than twenty books on consolation for bereaved Muslim parents were written in Egypt and Syria. It is believed that this genre bloomed as a result of the Black Plague, during which many parents lost all of their children at once.[8] The treatises are composed of hadith, accounts recorded in early Islam and attributed to the Prophet Muhammad and his followers.[9] These works often offered parents practical ways of coping with a child's death as a means of psychotherapy rather than religious philosophy.

Unlike the ancient Greeks and Romans, medieval Muslim parents reacted emotionally to the deaths of their children, a contradiction to Aries' claim that parents in the Middle Ages were indifferent to their children. The authors of these consolation treatises called for parents to demonstrate steadfastness or *sabr*.[10] Parents were called upon to restrain their emotions and to avoid protesting against "God's decree", and to show patience in the time of death. It is worth noting here that the "decree" refers to the death of an adult child while the consolation treatises referred to infant and child death.[11]

Authors of two such treatises in the fourteenth and fifteenth centuries related the story about a Muslim mother who postpones telling her husband of their son's death until they conceive again the following evening. The authors' intention for including the story is to praise the *sabr* of the bereaved mother. The story illustrates that the woman showed patience and was duly rewarded with the birth of another child.[12] Ancient and medieval sources frequently describe the sociobiological response of parents who conceive immediately after a child's death. This response is common in modern times as well and is discussed at length in Chapter 8. The Muslim treatises also describe a Jewish woman's experience losing two sons, although the reward for the woman's steadfastness is more supernatural. While her husband and his guests are enjoying a meal that she prepared for them, her two sons fell into a well and died. She hid their bodies in her room and did not tell her husband what had happened. When he inquired about the children, she simply stated that "They are in the house." She then seduced her husband. After, he asked about his sons again, and she gave the same reply. When he called for the children himself, they came out of the room and went to him. The woman then said "Glory be to God! They were both dead, and God quickened them as a reward for my steadfastness."[13]

The main purpose of the consolation treatises was to "channel the strong emotional reactions of bereaved parents into legitimate religious modes of mourning".[14] Many of the treatises spoke of rewards for patience and advice on how to control emotions when one is overcome with grief. The sheer scope and quantity of these treatises demonstrates the gravity of child death in the Middle Ages. While not the original purpose, these manuals offer historians and social researchers an indicator of the demographic repercussions of the plague and the corresponding suffering of parents during this time.

Poetry

Medieval Islam

Lamentation poems, often included in the medieval Muslim treatises, illustrated the psychological torment experiences by grieving parents. Frequently, the poetry spoke to the personal attributes of the child; intelligence and good character, for example. One such poem by Ibn Nubata states "'The child was small', they say, 'not so the grief for him,' say I".[15] Again, this statement echoes the common belief that young child, particularly under the age of three, should not be mourned.

Jan of Poland's Laments

Jan Kochanowski, a great Polish poet, wrote *Laments* when his two and a half year old daughter, Ursula, died in 1579. These nineteen poems begin as eulogy to her death, followed by lamentations expressing the depth of Jan's grief. The excerpt from Lament 1, below, exemplifies his denial of steadfastness. Like the other Laments that follow, it is an expression of unbearable grief.

> Help me to mourn my small girl, my dear daughter,
> Whom cruel Death tore up with such wild force
> Out of my life, it left me no recourse.

So the snake, when he finds a hidden nest
Of fledgling nightingales, rears and strikes fast
Repeatedly, while the poor mother bird
Tries to distract him with a fierce, absurd
Fluttering—but in vain! the venomous tongue
Darts, and she must retreat on ruffled wing.
"You weep in vain," my friends will say. But then,
What is not in vain, by God, in lives of men?
All is in vain! We play at blindman's buff
Until hard edges break into our path.
Man's life is error. Where, then, is relief?
In shedding tears or wrestling down my grief?[16]

Jan's series of poems conclude with a consolation and description of a dream in which he sees his daughter in the arms of his deceased mother. In the following Lament, the last, he is comforted by the knowledge that his daughter has eternal life and is protected from a potentially difficult adult life. This aggrieved father acknowledges the healing nature of time.

She ran her given course and did depart;
And if that course was brief, yet who can say
That she would have been happier to stay?
The ways of God are past our finding out,
Yet what He holds as good shall we misdoubt?
And when the spirit leaves us, it is vain
To weep so long; it will not come again…
That we should not lament when she hath done
A bitter turn, but thank her in that she
Hath held her hand from greater injury…Now,
master, heal thyself: time is the cure
For all.[17]

Lutheran Consolation Poetry in Modern Germany

Even after the plague's reach was extinguished, toward the end of Middle Ages, child mortality was extremely high in early modern Europe. It was very possible that a mother who bore over a dozen children outlived nearly all of them as well as her grandchildren, if there were any. Consolatory literature was prevalent among early modern German Lutherans. Martin Luther himself lost an infant and an adolescent, both females, and suffered greatly for the loss. The following excerpt of a letter Luther sent to a friend demonstrates his anguish. "My small daughter, my little Elisabeth has died. How strangely wretched it has left my spirit, almost like a woman's, so that I am moved by the pity of it, for I would never before have believed that fathers' spirits could grow so tender towards their children. Pray for me to the Lord, in whom I take my leave. Wittenberg, 1528, 5th August."[18]

Lutheran clergy began to write consolation manuals for bereaved parents as they came to realize that grief over the loss of a child, no matter how frequent the sorrowful event, was a natural response. Funerary poetry became common among the educated in seventeenth century Germany, particularly as a means of income. The poetry often became a part of a funeral booklet which also included the sermon, a biography of the deceased, and speeches and music from the funeral.[19]

During the reformation the Catholic concept of Purgatory, where the unbaptized soul would rest neither in heaven nor hell, was abandoned. Thus, the deceased could not be aided in their journey toward to heaven. Therefore, the focus, after the death of a child, was on comforting the living. The consolation books written at this time trained the parent in the proper amount of grief acceptable; that is, in moderation. They taught parents techniques for dealing with their sorrow and offered model prayers "in the hope that they will internalize and appropriate the arguments, putting them in a better position to cope with life's trials."[20] Additionally, the messages within poetry and consolation books, expressed by its Lutheran writers, focused on themes such as relieving parents from endless worry of the fate of their deceased children.

Yiddish Holocaust Lullabies

Often the genre of consolatory literature evolves in response to a series of tragic events. Yiddish lullabies were identified as surviving from Holocaust writings, with explicit themes of "persecution, death, abandonment, guilt and mourning."[21] Theses lullabies, often written in ghettos or camps in Europe, appear to have been composed and sung to help people cope with massive psychological trauma. Some authors were identified as parents of dead children, but others wrote to newly born, unborn, and orphaned children, as well as mothers and the Jewish people in general.[22] Some poems speak of the fear of the time. The following poem is a parent's appeal to a crying child:

> Here me, child-the sentry hovers
> Near us, so don't cry!
> He might shoot, if he discovers
> someone didn't die.[23]

Common themes in these poems are consolations to the child, who is either dead or likely will be soon, and who will soon be released from fear and want:

> Child, on the other side of the wall
> The ghetto is done with, once and for all;
> Somewhere a bird will sing in the sky,
> Shut forever your angel-eye
> Child, on the other side of the town
> no guns, no charged wire can be found;
> we'll dream a longtime, you and I,
> shut forever your angel-eye—
> husha, hushabye[24]

Nineteenth Century England and America

In nineteenth century England and America, child death was a predominant theme in both literature and poetry. Some of the most popular works included: *Stepping Heavenward* (1869), *The Empty Crib* (1873), *Agnes and the Key of Her Little Coffin* (1857), *Our Children in Heaven* (1870), and *Gates Ajar* (1868). *Gates Ajar* by Elizabeth Stuart Phelps was written in response to the aftermath of the Civil War.

As noted above, poems served to educate parents in appropriate mourning in addition to providing consolation; they advised parents not to weep as the child was "now [thought to be] an angel". In a poem written to a deceased child, Felicia Hemans explains that openly mourning and the use of funerary symbols were denied, even for a beloved child. "No bitter tears for thee…We rear no marble o'er thy tomb; No sculptured image there shall mourn".[25]

Despite, the belief that expressions of grief should be tempered, colonial mothers (and indeed, mothers everywhere) insisted that it was biology, carrying the child for nine months and subsequently nursing for as many as three years, which entitled her to mourn. While in the above poem, Felicia Hemans advises steadfastness, she later says to her grieving sister in a letter "I can feel deeply for the sorrow you communicate to me; it is one which Heaven has yet graciously spared me; but the imagination…has often brought all the sufferings of that particular bereavement before me, with a vividness from which I have shrunk almost in foreboding terror. And I have too those sick and weary yearnings for the dead…"[26]

During the eighteenth century the Quakers in Philadelphia counseled parents to find consolation in resignation to "God's will". Mourning was a process through which the living "took stock of their own spiritual health" and prepared for their own death. While parents were also urged to keep "due distance" from infants in order to protect themselves from the grief that the child's death would bring, parents, mothers in particular, found respite in a new form of consolation literature beyond the emotionally charged poetry that stemmed from this time. Lowry Wister, an eighteenth century Philadelphia mother, provided us with an example of consolation literature, likely meant to be private, in the form of a diaries and letters to her sister and children. Shortly after her three year old son's unexpected death from small pox, Wister set out to describe the events and her attendant feelings about her young child's demise. In her narrative Wister does not discuss the preparation of the body, burial or any other mourning rituals, which are often public. Instead, she only writes about the grief she experiences. But by expressing her grief and even questioning the doctor's choice of treatment for her son, she is retaliating against the notion of resignation. By "textualizing her loss" she memorializes the bond she had with her son.[27]

By basis of comparison, Wister's twenty year old daughter Sarah wrote a more typical example of consolation which was tinged with the concept of resignation: "in the full bloom of health and beauty it pleas'd the Lord of heaven to call him from a world of woe and misery in to the regions of happiness…" Contrasting this with Mrs. Wister's remembrance of her son's last words "mamy where is thee.'…[these words] everlastingly engraven on my heart", illustrates the private realm of a mother's grief versus societal expectations. These writings helped to support new modes of allowing other women to similarly grieve.[28]

Modern Consolation

Consolation literature met a need when people did not openly discuss maternal grief. In the 1970s several books were published that addressed the loss of a baby or child, as well as the mother's need to express, and have acknowledged, the grief that attends such a loss. Simonds and Katz Rothman, comparing these books and other consolation literature (self-help books, clippings from women's magazines, poetry, newsletters) from the 1970s to poetry of the nineteenth century, ask: why was women's grief addressed in the nineteenth century and not at other times? One explanation is that women's grief was valued because it "could be used to respond to the excesses of industrialization".[29] In essence women and clergy men were working to "validate and glorify death in America" toward a greater good.[30]

In an example from 1900, the "Baby's Drawer", by Anonymous, a mother describes the joy of her son's birth, the event of his death and her subsequent grief and the clothing he will never wear:

Ah, the radiant summer morning,
So full of a mother's joy!
Thank God he is fair and perfect,
My beautiful, new-born boy.
Let him wear the pretty white garments
I wrought while sitting apart;

Many and Many an evening
I sit since my baby came,
Saying, "what do the angels call him?"
For he died without a name.

Sit while the hours are waning,
And the house is all at rest,
And fancy a baby nestling
Close to my aching breast[31]

Sometimes poetry reflects a parent's regrets. In "A Silent House" by Pearl Eyetinge, in 1988, the mother laments "How oft I stilled the noisy chatter…and wished the song and play would cease, or prayed for just one moment's peace…. Ah! God! That I may be forgiven, And meet my little child in Heaven."[32]

In some of the more recent literature of the 1970s, the insensitivity to mothers who have had a miscarriage or stillbirth is acknowledged. Ignorant outsiders try to console the aggrieved mother by expressing statements such as: "at least you didn't know it well" or "you can always have another", as if these souls were fleeting thoughts caught and released, never to be visited again. Other poems describe the anguish a mother suffers during a miscarriage. Marion J. Helz Perry, in 1983, writes "I dreamed of a baby…Just at the time you would have been born…Why did that dream have to come when you should have." In "The Lost Children" Barbara Crooker describes how miscarried children pervade lives of their parents. The loss is timeless:

The ones we never speak of-
Miscarried, unborn,
Removed by decree

Taken too soon, crossed over.
They slip red mittens in our hands,
Smell of warm wet wool,
Are always out of sight.
We glimpse them on escalators,

Over the shoulders of dark-haired women;
They return to us in dreams.
We hold them, as they evanesce;
We never speak their names
How many children do you have?
Two, we answer, thinking three…
They are always with us

The lost children come to us at night
And whisper in the shells of our ears.
They are waving goodbye on school buses,
Separated from us in stadiums,
Lost in shopping malls;
At the beach they disappear
behind the first wave.[33]

Another poem, from 1990, represents the voice of a pregnant mother comforting her friend who had experienced ten miscarriages and a recent stillbirth. In this poem, "Giving away the Layette", the grieving mother gives away the baby clothes that she has collected but were never worn. The poem concludes with a consolation by the author: "We will sit by you…For however long it takes. Your labor is not yet over. Mine will be light."[34]

From these selections we can ascertain that while death of the young was frequent, grief was a natural and expected reaction. In ancient societies the literature indicates that there was a line that must not be crossed when it came to self-restraint; grief must be commensurate with the child's age at death. Later, in the twentieth century, it became much more widely accepted to grieve openly.

10

Visual Representations of Child Death

Artwork and Photographs

Visual representations of deceased children served a purpose far beyond that of recording an image. They often also reflected societies', and more specifically parents', attitudes toward death. Additionally, the function of these works was also to console or facilitate the grieving process.[1] Ever since early Modern history, artists had painted pictures of dead children laid out for their funerals. The evidence left to us through photographs, paintings, and cemetery monuments provides a romanticized perspective of child death. For example, the Victorian practice of having a posthumous portrait of a dead child painted to represent a living child, while displaying it with photographs of the child's corpse, illustrates the complex dynamic of acceptance and denial within Victorian society.[2]

Van Setten observes that in the Netherlands, and possibly in the Western world in general, early nineteenth century people started to give more attention to the consolation of grieving parents. During the seventeenth and eighteenth centuries few traces of guilt could be found in Dutch expressions of grief. This is unusual because most grieving parents express regret at what they could have done (e.g., sought medical help, baptized an infant so that he would not linger forever in purgatory). Therefore, the shift to artistic representations of dead children and their grieving parents in the nineteenth century is significant.[3] Van Setten also observes that there was an abundance of consolatory literature, particularly in the form of poetry.

Representation of Children in Art

In *Imagining Childhood,* Erika Langmuir, referring to pharaonic Egypt in particular, notes that commemoration with funeral images of children is rare in the ancient world. When children's images can be found, it is "prospective—a means of attaining immortality in Osiris' divine realm, that symbolizes both death and fertility." Further, she notes that Classical and Hellenistic art uses children to commemorate the mother or grandmother, rather than the child itself. In one example of a figure found on a gravestone, a woman holds an infant in one arm, while entertaining it with a toy or figure with the other hand. The inscription alludes to the fact that she is the grandmother who predeceased the child; they are now together. On a second or third century Greek stele an image of a dead toddler waves to his mother as he begins a journey on the River Styx. The mother's grief is evident in her stature, although the child does not appear to understand his fate. While the image depicts the mythological journey of the soul, Langmuir notes that the intention is to express both individuality and maternal love, and to offer consolation. Unlike Egyptian art, Greek art determines to express emotion in addition to communicating a story.[4]

The representation of children in Roman funerary art transformed from the first to fourth centuries. While historians ask "What does the evidence left behind by artists prove?" the answer may lie in the artists' interpretation of society. On tomb reliefs children in the first century were seen in a familial context, depicted clearly as children. Later, however, they began to be represented as little adults on funerary alters, perhaps donning a military cloak, indicating hopes for what a son would have been had he survived. One particular portrait depicts two infants being suckled by a hind, yet portrayed like men with togas and scrolls. Other ways of honoring children was to associate them with gods or goddess. In the second century, as burials replaced cremation, panels allowed for child-centered images of boys and girls playing together or even death bed scenes. Interestingly, boys were depicted in scenes relating to the ideal of what they might achieve, where girls were shown in a scene at death, as if asleep. Explanations for these changes in representation can be explained, in part, by the adoption of Christianity.[5] Much of ancient art depicting children showed them as engaged in play. These images worked to impress upon parents that children will be eternally absorbed in the "little things".

Roman children's sarcophagi often mirrored that of adults, albeit on a smaller scale, although some motifs included children playing games, or racing chariots. Some scenes are described as *conclamatio* which show the mourning of a dead child. In one example of such a work a child's biography is illustrated: he is nursed by his mother in one scene, his father appears to educate him in another, in one of the last he is an older child driving a chariot. In another *conclamatio* the cycle of an infant's life is displayed: he is depicted as a newborn, then shown moving through the milestones of toddlerhood. At the end of the cycle the infant's family is shown retreating in a carriage led by a *putto*. The sarcophagus is flanked by two torches, which may be symbolic of the practice of burying children at night. In another example, a deceased child is laid out on the couch. The scene depicts someone recording the death, which Langmuir notes only occurs on children's sarcophagi, especially those of girls. *Conclamatio* scenes which depicted life as it would actually be scene (no flying *putti*) are intended to portray an "eternal present". *Conclamatio* later inspired images of dead children in European art. They are portrayed as members of the family or as angels watching protectively over surviving parents and siblings.

Consequently, Sebastian Brant, during the Northern Renaissance in 1502, published an illustrated edition of *Aeneid,* which depicted Aeneas' descent in to the underworld in Book VI. The representation of the weeping souls of infants plunged to their death was disturbing to Brant. Instead the publisher chose to follow the lead of Greek sculptors, and depicted the children as "unconscious of their fate"; swaddled, being cuddled and nursed, and fiendishly engaging with fellow young inhabitants of the underworld, oblivious to the life they no longer occupy.[6]

Paintings of children often included a dead sibling shown as though still alive. The Graham children, painted by William Hogarth in the mid-eighteenth century, are one such example. Symbols of death pervade the painting: a cherub, still life of fruit, flowers at the feet of the child, and an hour glass and clock above him (stopped at the time of death) signal to the viewer that the child is indeed dead. Flowers symbolize fragility, while painted fruit never rots—the presence of these items is a consolation to the family that their grief will "be sublimated". Similarly, Nicolaes Maes portrayed dead children as Ganymede, the Trojan boy who was stolen away by Jupiter disguised as an eagle.[7]

Memorial Photography

Where burial and cremation omitted the dead from daily reminders to the living, memorial photographs served as proof of a child's existence. Memorial, or post-mortem, photography is a visual method of illustrating responses to death and differences in mourning practices between cultures. Postmortem photographs of children were common in the nineteenth and twentieth centuries, in both America and Europe, when child mortality was at staggering levels, and it was not unusual for parents to lose all of their children to small pox, diphtheria, or another epidemic. While post-mortem paintings were frequently created for the wealthy, post-mortem photography was an affordable means by which the middle and lower classes could memorialize loved ones. Quite often the memorial photograph was the first and only image ever taken of a person. These images were usually put on display in the home, or made into jewelry and distributed to family members. In modern times, as the incidence of child death is uncommon, the practice might be considered unusual (although renewed interest in this type of photography has now made it more widely accepted). These photographs were (and are) a normal part of the grieving process. Memorial photography was very much an art form. During the Victoria era, for example, death was beautifully depicted as "restful sleep". The practice allowed mourners to visually preserve the dead, while also distancing themselves; a natural and healthy part of the grieving process.[8]

These photographs also served as means by which to examine how mourning practices have evolved. For example, in the nineteenth century mourning clothes and jewelry were often black or purple, and women wore veils over their faces. In the second stage of mourning, the veil is lifted and non-black jewelry could be worn. Subsequently, some remnants would be worn to indicate that one was still grieving. Sometimes it was not sufficient for a peaceful photo to be taken as remembrance of the child. While images including both parents were rare, one particular photograph titled "Mother and father with dead daughter, useless medicine bottles on the table" was presumably taken to illustrate failed medical intervention as well as parental mourning. Often photographs including parents attempted to illustrate parents' grief by showing them holding the dead child. Until the fear of contagious diseases ended the practice, it was common practice for parents to bring deceased children to the photographer for these photographs.[9]

Usually children were depicted as sleeping, although in the late 1800s the photographer R.B. Whittaker advertised the ability to photograph a dead child as both "awake" and "asleep" by painting the eyes open. Children were often portrayed angelically, surrounded by loved toys, and objects symbolizing death such as a clock, wilted flowers, or a willow tree. Typically, parents wanted to create a beautiful and serene setting. A common advertising slogan for memorial photographers in the nineteenth century was "secure the shadow, ere the substance fade".[10]

When there were siblings, they were often called upon to pose with their dead brothers or sisters. In modern times we might shield the very young from death; in the nineteenth century, however, children were taught to fear death by both their parents and the church. They were often present when family members died in their homes and during funeral preparations.[11]

In some cases photographers were summoned to capture the images of dying children. One such photograph, titled "Woman cradling her dying son", shows the mother holding her fading child while he takes his last breaths. The photograph is exhibited next to another in which the mother is visibly bereaved. Clearly the photographs were taken minutes apart—after her son has died. In another photograph a woman is seen holding her five or six year old child, which was unusual because older children were usually laid out on a couch or bed. Burns interprets the pose of the mother as unwilling to release her daughter. In a similar photograph, a mother kept her daughter, preserved with ice, from being buried for nine days (children were typically buried the day after they died). As these photographs were intended to illustrate familial bonds, parents' inclusion in the image is "an admittance of loss and final separation". In another photograph, intended as a means by which to publically demonstrate, and therefore recognize the effect of child death, four grieving women pose with their faces obscured by handkerchiefs into which they are apparently weeping.[12] An image of a mother holding a photograph of her dead child, instead of the child itself, demonstrates the significance of memorial photography. Stanley Burns argues that this image indicates the "authority of photography as representation of the real."[13]

Another genre of memorial photography attempted to show the dead child as alive by propping up the corpse and opening its eyes.[14] In some cases, photographs were taken of mothers caring for their sick and dying children. The reasons for the emergence of this type of photography are unclear, although one reason may be a form of denial of the death of the child.[15] Another may be the fulfilling of a wish by parents to have the photo that had never been taken when the child was alive.[16] It is interesting to note that disabled children were also often lovingly photographed, which indicates a contradiction to the often held belief that parents of past centuries were unable or unwilling to love children with special needs.

In the 1920s the practice of professional postmortem photography faded, although some ethnic groups continued the custom. Informal photographing of dead children occurs today however. Since parents have taken over as family photographers, many of those photographs have not made their way into the public domain of archives.[17] In recent years, hospitals have begun to record children at their death, whether stillborn infants or fully developed children. Organizations, such as "Now I Lay Me Down To Sleep", have been established to offer pre- and postmortem photographs free of charge to grieving parents.[18] The sessions are conducted sensitively and with professionalism. The photographs, while often difficult to view, are a beautiful memorial to the deceased child and a loving illustration of the intimate relationship between parent and child, whether just born or a firmly established member of the family. Most recently some artists have expanded the genre to include drawings or paintings based on postmortem photographs (as some parents prefer an artistic rendition of an image of the deceased child), drawings of a preterm infants projected to look as they would if they had survived to full term, and videos. These images have been indicated as an aid to the grieving process. As Burns notes, these images allow loved ones to grieve their dead at a healthy distance.

11 Infanticide and Child Sacrifice

An Overview

In each chapter of this book infanticide has been discussed within various historical and sociological contexts. Accordingly, Williamson, in *Infanticide and the Value of Life*, succinctly states that "Infanticide has been practiced on every continent and by people on every level of cultural complexity, from hunter gatherers to high civilizations, including our own ancestors. Rather than being an exception, then, it has been the rule."[1] The purpose of the following chapter is to provide background on infanticide and child sacrifice, while also addressing the complexities that cause different cultures to accept these practices.

The historical literature is rich with examples of parents murdering their own children. Women often committed infanticide in order to hide an affair (or otherwise inappropriate sexual relationship), avoid being ostracized socially or professionally, or because of their inability to care for the child. In the modern developed world, given the legalization of abortion in most countries, access to social services, and options for adoption, most women who commit infanticide are teenagers.

In the twentieth and twenty-first centuries, as courts have come to understand how women were affected by childbirth and postpartum depression, mothers who commit infanticide have been treated more compassionately than in centuries prior. In 1922 the criminal charge for infanticide was reduced from a capital crime to manslaughter, and generally included only infants killed within the first year of life. People who killed older children were still charged with murder, and usually punished with life in prison. Prior to this time unmarried women were the target of laws against infanticide, in part to punish them for immoral behavior. When a child's death was caused by a parent's neglect, which was considered indirect infanticide, the punishment was less clear.[2] What is compelling about infanticide practiced from the eighteenth century to the present is that it is almost always performed by females. Females rarely kill. In fact, crime is largely a male phenomenon. When women do kill, it is people close to them: husbands, boyfriends, and children.[3]

Questions have arisen about many prehistoric and ancient burials as to whether they are a result of sex selected infanticide/sacrifice, or due to other social or biological causes. Infanticide is suspected in places where a disproportionate amount of female infants are found. In some cultures, however, sacrifice of best-loved or first-born sons is common, and in these societies a large amount of male infants might be found. In matrilineal societies, as in Jamaica for example, females are highly valued for their ability to provide economically. But they are only valuable if they can retain their wealth throughout their lives. In cultures where dowries are paid for daughters, families with more sons than daughters generally inherit more wealth. Scott argues that since the 1980s, where females have more independence and success, women do not require husbands to have children. They may retain their birth names and often out-achieve, academically, men in many subjects. Accordingly, the birth of daughters is often met with joy and pride—particularly in well developed nations where women's rights are held in esteem.[4]

Causes and Reasons for Infanticide

Maria Piers, writing in 1978, tells the story of how a college class of city sewer workers revealed how common it was to discover babies in the sewers; apparently an unexceptional place for abandoning newborn infants since the invention of sewers in ancient Rome. Piers assumes that the mothers were poor, uneducated, young, and unfeeling toward their infants, and who perceived their babies to be strange and despicable objects on par with detritus since they did not choose to place the child with an adoption agency, or abandon the baby in a safer place.

Poverty, among the many causes articulated by Piers, is one of the main reasons parents kill their children. In the barrios of Latin America some parents will maim their children to the point of crippling so that the children can beg. Apparently, crippling is less sinful than using birth control, or performing infanticide or abortion. Within these poverty-stricken areas, where large families are the norm, the seventh or eighth child is often doomed to starvation and neglect, particularly if they are female or dark-skinned. In the barrios the position of "infant undertaker" is prominent, given the large number of funerals for babies.

Piers also notes that infanticide occurs when large numbers of people are "violently uprooted" whether by man-made disasters, such as wars, or natural disasters, like floods. In these circumstances a newborn, with less attachment to the parent and no knowledge of his or her fate, is chosen to bear a slow death by neglect as direct infanticide is often too difficult carry out. Massive infanticide has always occurred among famine and hopelessness as humans become self-centered for survival—a child might be considered competition for food and resources. As the weakest member of the community they are at risk.[5]

At the root of many of these causes, Piers argues, is the view that the child is a thing; she terms this "basic strangeness". Basic strangeness is in some part a result of the inability to bond with a child. A neglected woman, without a positive example of a maternal figure, and hungry for both a mother figure and affection, might look to have a baby to fill that need. Yet, when the baby is not happy, quiet, and loveable, she may become impatient and unable to provide the unconditional love an unpredictable infant needs. Parenting humans is difficult, with a steep learning curve. It requires patience, maturity and flexibility. Here is where there is potential for a human parent to become either an excellent nurturer or a murder. In general, highly taxing incidental (last straw) experiences can turn a loving parent into a monster or a murderer.[6]

Disability as a Reason for Infanticide

Some historians have argued that children born with deformities are often targets of infanticide and sacrifice. In some respects, this is the case in modern society as well; severely disabled children, whose deformity might be detected in the early fetal stages, may often be prevented from being born through selective abortion. Archaeological evidence, however, does not always support the fact that deformed and disabled children were always candidates for infanticide. Even in the Middle Ages the disabled were accepted members of society. For example, special drinking pots adapted for child with cleft palates in the Middle Ages have been excavated recently. Additionally, in Chapter 2, I note the case in which a disabled child was buried, with care, with a typically-developed child, providing no evidence that there was differential burial treatment for those who were born with deformities. Even in ancient Rome, where many cases of infanticide have been uncovered, none of the supposed victims were revealed to have had deformities.[7]

Law and Punishment for Infanticide

In the late 1990s a surge of abandoned infants in the United States prompted law makers to enact Safe Haven laws in which each state allowed parents to relinquish unharmed infants to the authorities, "no questions asked", within seven days of birth without fear of legal action being taken against them. It is not uncommon to see a sign with a stylized illustration of an infant and the words "Safe Haven" in the vicinity of hospitals, police precincts, and firehouses to promote this law. Unfortunately, infanticide still occurs at the rate of about eighty-five per year.

The Safe Haven law is a counterpoint to the Basil decree in which, in the fifteenth century, a woman abandoning her child at a town hall (or another public place) would be thrown into the Rhine. Presumably this punishment was given because of the lack of wet nurses at orphanages, which might have ultimately caused the child's demise anyway.[8] Other laws established to punish women actually encouraged mothers to kill their newborns. For example, King Frederick William I of Prussia issued an edict in 1723 against unmarried women who had concealed their pregnancies. If they then claimed to have given birth to a stillborn child, the concealment was considered a sign of intentional murder.[9]

Preceding their present iteration, laws on infanticide in both England and New England emerged between 1558 and 1803. While the act was condemned, little was done to stifle it. As in Prussia, concealment of a pregnancy, which ultimately resulted in a stillbirth, indicated intent to murder a child. It was not a felony, however, if the birth of a stillborn child to an unwed mother were concealed to avoid penalties or social isolation. Comparing court cases of infanticide in the sixteenth and seventeenth centuries with those in the eighteenth century, Hoffer and Hull traced the development of laws against infanticide within the context of changing perspectives of children, parents, and sex. Eventually, these laws resulted in very low conviction rates and brief prison sentences.[10]

Infanticide was common among poor, unwed mothers. The authorities looking down at these women, perceived them as having loose sexual morals. In Colonial America giving birth to an illegitimate child was a crime, and was punished with a lifetime of indentured servitude, which encouraged women to give birth secretly and, if a child were stillborn, bury the body surreptitiously. If the birth and subsequent secret burial were revealed, the woman was automatically assumed guilty of infanticide.[11] Unsurprisingly, the social and economic environment compelled these unmarried mothers to get rid of unplanned children. Therefore, social inequality, perceptions of sexuality, and standards propagated by religious leaders and lawmakers, in part, caused the epidemic of child murder which they simultaneously prosecuted. Further, in England cases of infanticide and witchcraft were often conflated. Sometimes one crime would be invented to explain the other.[12]

In medieval England few cases of infanticide were prosecuted by the courts, and when they were, rarely did coroner inquests lead to the determination of infanticide as a cause of death. One notable case involved the "one hundred of Chippenham", who were fined for letting Basilia of Wroxhall escape after she had thrown her infant son in a ditch only to have a dog retrieve the body, dragging it through the town. Other western European societies reacted differently to infanticide. For example, between 1500 and 1750 Nuremburg put eighty-seven women to death for the crime.[13]

A Brief History of Infanticide in Different Cultures and Time Periods

From prehistory to modern society, abandonment leading to death by exposure has been the most common method of infanticide. Newborns are the most susceptible to infanticide and were (and still are) usually smothered right after birth or abandoned. As noted previously, in many cultures infanticide tends to demonstrate favoring of one sex. For example, among Neolithic groups between fifteen and fifty percent of births resulted in infanticide. The wide variation in percentages is explained by the difficulties in determining whether children were victims of infanticide or had died of natural deaths (discussed further in Chapter 2).[14] Divale, however, found that in eighty-six hunter-gather societies where infanticide was practiced there was a gender ratio of 1.38 to 1, in favor of males, whereas in societies where it was not practiced the ratio was 1 to 1.[15] One explanation for this disparity is that some burial practices may have been reserved for specific genders of infants. Further, while female infanticide was more widely practiced, there have been episodes of male infanticide recorded in history. The Rendille in Kenya, for example, kill baby boys in order to limit the amount of potential male cattle owners; cattle being an essential resource. In Israel one hundred newborns were found in a Roman sewer under a bath house. Of those who had testable DNA, fourteen males and five females were identified. This was unusual in that infants were usually carefully buried at the time. Simon Mays hypothesizes that females may have been bred for prostitution by their prostitute mothers, which may have generated male infanticide.[16]

In ancient societies attempts to prevent infanticide were sometimes addressed with legislation. The Twelve Tables of Roman law stated that it was the duty of the patriarch of the family to decide whether newborns should be raised or destroyed, particularly if the child were visibly deformed. Ultimately, the adoption of Christianity in Rome caused the practice to abate as The Council of Constantinople declared infanticide illegal. Despite these laws it was not uncommon for baby girls to be exposed.[17]

Less infanticide was recorded during the Middles Ages, although it still occurred at staggering rates. Overlaying while nursing was a frequent cause of death among infants. The suspiciously high mortality rate indicates that overlaying may have been purposeful, whether by mother or wet nurse. As noted in Chapter 5, floods of children were abandoned in the Middle Ages. Wishful mothers, assuming their child to be a changeling, abandoned unwanted or sickly children, returning later in hopes that the child was reverted to health. When foundling homes were established to address the rash of infanticide and abandonment, children brought to these homes had between an eighty and one hundred percent chance of dying.

The Koran prohibits infanticide, although prior to the adoption of Islam in Arabian societies, the practice was used as a method of birth control called *wa'd.* It was practiced in cases of poverty, as a sacrifice, or upon the birth of a girl—who might have been buried alive if the father felt her death was warranted.[18] Sometimes a passive form of exsanguination, by not tying the umbilical cord, might have been used to kill an unwanted newborn female. In a dramatic show of desperation, a father might hold his infant daughter in one hand, and with a knife in the other, threaten to kill her unless some man took her for his wife.[19]

In early medieval China, Marco Polo noted that the Chinese exposed their children and, much like in current times, often killed females. When female babies were born they might be put into a bucket of cold water that stood waiting at the place birth, just in case. In the late 1800s, however, Chinese emperors began to issue warnings and make concerted efforts to end infanticide of girls. Orphanages were established in order to address the needs of families. In present day China, the One Child policy has contributed to abandonment, gender-selected abortion, and infanticide—all illegal. Children who ultimately end up in orphanages have a very high chance of dying. Children who are disabled in particular are often neglected. The documentary "The Dying Room" illustrates the unjust manner in which these children live and die. Infanticide in ancient China is discussed extensively in Chapter 3.

The samurai of the Tokugawa period (1615 to 1860) did not marry until age thirty, and found it unacceptable to have more than three children. Abortion was frequent if families became too large, or if the birth of daughters was too frequent. In Feudal Japan victims of infanticide were smothered when wet paper was placed on the baby's mouth and nose. The Japanese called infanticide *mabiki* (weeding an overcrowded garden), which occurred until the early twentieth century.[20] During the famine of 1783 cannibalism was prevalent. Those who died were eaten immediately by survivors. Those who perished from starvation, however, decayed too quickly to be consumed. In one village, for example, a man who already lost his wife and one child asked a neighbor to kill his remaining son with a sword so that he may be eaten before dying of starvation, in exchange for sharing the "meat". The father then turned the sword on the neighbor to avenge the death of his son and have double the quantity of meat.[21]

In South Asia infanticide of females was also common, especially those who were illegitimate. They were offered up as wives to anyone who might take them upon birth or immediately killed with a knife. In present day rural India the practice continues, although it is illegal.[22] Further, due to the rise in poverty, in Pakistan newborn babies are increasingly abandoned. In the year 2010 alone, 1,210 babies were found dead and inappropriately discarded.[23]

Infant and Child Sacrifice

Children were often selected over adults for sacrifice as they were deemed more pure and free from sin, thus closer to god. Reasons for sacrifice included appeasing war gods to salve illness, or to overcome illness or infertility. A child's blood was considered "magic milk". While in both hemispheres of the earth infanticide was regularly practiced regardless of the legitimacy of a child, in many societies it went unpunished or undetected; in comparison some scholars contend that child sacrifice was relatively rare.[24]

Sacrifice is not a direct reflection of a parent's love for a child. Rather it is an expression of deeply held beliefs. In fact many victims of sacrifice were the best-loved children. Among the Phoenicians, for example, mothers could be heard wailing for their babies as they were incinerated. Some women were paid to sacrifice their children in place of those originally selected. Sacrifice victims were usually infants, male, and could be rich or poor, depending upon whether it was the dedicant's child or one bought expressly for sacrifice. Sacrifice often required considerable planning and assistance. Carthaginian parents added their names to markers indicating that they had fulfilled their responsibility to their deity.[25]

Modern societies might deem sacrifice as cruel or as evidence of detachment from one's children. It is not just the killing of children, but the "dispos[al] of infants and young children who had been fully accepted into what they saw as the social and legal unit of the family" that is disturbing to people. While there is a temptation to judge sacrificial acts by modern standards or even by those of ancient or Christian Rome, it is important to consider what these rituals meant at the time. It was the suffering of the families who offered their children that was the gift that would mollify the gods. Sacrifice also "binds the family to the state' through the family's loss and the state's gain", indicating that children did not belong to their parents but to the community and the gods. The practices of Spartan parents illustrates this link between family and state: at the age of seven Spartans sent their boys to state-run houses to prepare to be warriors, although Spartan infants were only killed if they were deemed unable to live up to the state's physical demands.[26]

Later, animals were increasingly used in addition to or in lieu of infants; however, other researchers note that as the Phoenicians urbanized, child sacrifice actually increased. In the tophets, the ritual burial spaces where infants were sacrificed until Rome destroyed Carthage during the last Punic War in 146 BC, 20,000 burial urns were found. While this number sounds like an exceedingly high amount of children, it represents an average of about two sacrifices per week (or one hundred per year). Compared to the Aztecs, who sacrificed 20,000 people per year, this relatively small number does not indicate mass sacrifice, but a Phoenician ritual to regularly fulfill a vow to the gods. Appeasement of the god *Molech* by child sacrifice is indicated by the name *mlk ba'al* on a child's stelae, while the inscription of the word *mlk 'mr* was used when an animal was sacrificed. Some researchers argue as to whether these tophets really do indicate sacrifice, but others point out that children were found to be buried in shallow graves in non-sacrificial cemeteries, while infants buried in tophets were cremated and placed in non-funerary pottery.[27] As noted in Chapter 3, research published in 2013 confirms that these tophets were evidence of sacrifice.

Among the Inca in Peru *capacocha* (human sacrifice) was practiced with young children, but not with infants. Usually children who were sacrificed were buried with miniature animals molded from precious metals. Death was a metaphor for planting seeds. Therefore, the sacrifice of children is connected to fertility and production. Older children were chosen for sacrifice as they were considered old enough to talk to dead ancestors so that they might ask for qualities such as strength for the community.

Unlike the Inca, the Moche, an earlier culture of the north coast of Peru, appeared to have sacrificed infants in a plaza of the Huaca de la Luna, a ceremonial center for the Moche. In one instance, three infants were found underneath a large group of sacrificed men who had been captured in battle and killed during *el Nino* weather events (such as heavy rains and flooding). This indicated that the ritual killing of the infants preceded that of the adults. Like other excavations that appear to be sacrificial sites, it is possible that the burial of the children, whose skeletons were missing their heads, might be reflective of an enactment of a scene from Moche pottery. The pottery illustrates the decapitation of an infant as it is born from a whistling woman. Therefore, the infants might have died naturally and been buried in this sacrificial space because they were considered to have special qualities. Further, the babies did not have the same knife marks on their vertebrae that the decapitated adults had. Additionally, perhaps to reflect the Moche whistling woman, one of the infants was found with a whistle in each hand. Whether the children themselves were sacrificed or not, they were buried in a sacrificial context as part of a larger gift to the gods to protect them from the effects of *el Nino*.

Infants found at the Roman Empire temple at Springhead, Kent in Britain provide strong evidence of sacrifice when compared to infants buried elsewhere in the site. Two infants, one of which was decapitated, were found buried in opposite corners in the foundation of a building. The six month old babies were placed on their sides in a flexed (as opposed to a more natural fetal) position. Beneath these two infants were two more children (where, again, only one infant was decapitated) of the same age, which appeared to be ceremonially buried about ten years previously. The decapitation indicates a "link with the Roman-Celtic ritual of separation of the head from the whole" which was typically expressed through sculpture or animals. Some historians have argued that perhaps the infants were physically deformed or otherwise unwanted children. Malformed children, typically candidates for infanticide in some cultures, might have been diverted toward the purpose of sacrifice instead. Conversely, these may have been best loved children offered up for sacrifice.[28]

In India children were killed for economic and spiritual reasons. Bathing in a child's blood was considered a remedy for disease. If a woman was having difficulty becoming pregnant, or in order to produce a healthy child after the loss of an ill child, she was directed to bathe in the blood of a murdered child. In another example, in order to bless their journey, the Banjarilu, travelling traders of southern India, would bury a small child to his shoulders in the sand, and then traders would drive their bullocks over the child until he was dead. They believed that the amount of success they had on their journey was commensurate with the thoroughness of the trampling. Sacrifice was performed until 1800 in Saugor when the governor put an end to the practice, despite the objections of Brahmin priests. Near this city young men would throw themselves from the hills on to the rocks below in order to fulfill their mothers' vows to the god of destruction. Ironically, this vow was made in order to overcome barrenness.[29]

The prevalence of infanticide and sacrifice troubles many historians when making the connection between loving attitudes towards children and the high incidence of infant mortality. Mark Golden notes that modern studies of women who have chosen to have an abortion at some time in their lives revealed that many of those women planned to have children in the future. Thus, he makes the connection between infanticide and failed attempts at birth control; infant exposure and infanticide in ancient or pre-modern history do not necessarily emanate from hostility toward children.[30]

Notes

Introduction

1. Aries, 1973, p. 57.
2. See for example, Wilson, 1984.
3. See Hanawalt,1993 and Wilson,1984 for example.
4. Hanawalt, 1993, introduction.
5. Ibid.
6. Shorter quoted in Pollock, 1983, p. 3.
7. Pollock, 1983.
8. Quoted in Pollock, 1983, p. 7. For a more extensive review of the family history literature in support of positive parental attitudes toward children see Pollock, 1983 pages 1–32.
9. Quoted in deMause, 1974.
10. Ibid.
11. Slater, 1977, p. 15.
12. CIA World Fact Book.
13. Wilson, 1984.
14. Hanawalt, 1993.
15. Rawson, 2003.
16. Golden, 1988.

17. Gil'adi, 1992.
18. Ibid.
19. Rawson, 2003.
20. For example Aries, 1973; Scheper-Hughes, 1992. Scheper-Hughes presents a more complicated view of this phenomenon in her ethnography of women in Brazil, discussed more fully in Chapter 6.
21. Stone, 1977.
22. Goldberg, 1977 p. 235.
23. Van Setten, 1999 p. 8.
24. deMause, 1974, p. 17.
25. Wilson, 1984.

Chapter 1

1. Dye and Smith, 1986.
2. United Nations, 2011.
3. Ibid.
4. CDC 2011.
5. Dye and Smith, 1986. While this two-sided message was likely delivered to mothers worldwide, the phenomenon is noted widely by Dye and Smith. In general, however, it is neglect and ignorance that has been recorded as the underlying cause of infant death where it has been intolerably high in nearly every region of the world across time periods, with few notable exceptions (discussed later in this chapter).
6. Buchan, quoted in deMause.
7. Russell, 2007. In her NY Times article, Russell discusses the lack of reporting on children, particularly baby girls, placed in orphanages and available for adoption. Munro, 1996, discusses the fact that some mortality rates ranged from 59% to as high as 73% in Fujian, Shaanxi, Guangxi, and Henan, China.
8. Iwaniec, 2004.
9. Reid, et al., 2006.
10. Jordan, 1987.
11. Fildes, 1986.
12. Ibid.
13. Jordon, 1987.
14. Fidelis, 1986.
15. deMause, 1974, asserts that some infants were sent to wet nurses expressly for the purpose of being murdered, whether by beating, neglect or overdose of Laudanum (to quiet a crying baby) among many other causes.
16. Breschi, Manfredini, Pozzi, 2004.
17. Oris et al., 2004.

18. Ibid.
19. Razzel and Spence, 2004.
20. Edvinsson, 2004.
21. Schmelz, 1971.
22. Derosas, 2003.
23. Ali et al., 2003.
24. Guha-Sapir and Gijsbert van Panhuis, 2004.
25. Saha and van Soest, 2011.
26. Wood, Magno de Carvalho and Guimaraes Horta, 2010.
27. Reher and Sanz Gimeno, 2004.
28. Ibid.
29. Saha and van Soest, 2011.
30. Colon and Colon, 2001.
31. Preston and Haines, 1991.
32. Dunn in de Mause, 1974, p. 392.
33. deMause, 1974.
34. Colon and Colon, 2001.
35. Sundin,1996.
36. Ibid.
37. Kent, 1991, p. 57.

Chapter 2

1. Potter et al., 2011.
2. Murphy, 2011, Sarah Tarlow urges archaeologists to consider emotional values in archaeology, for example.
3. Derevenski, 1994.
4. See chapter 7, and the reference to Indians at the San Francisco Mission.
5. Raczek, 2003.
6. Colon and Colon, 2001, p. 4.
7. Ibid., p. 5.
8. Roveland, 2000.
9. Colon and Colon, 2001.
10. Scott, 1999.
11. Zagorska, 2008, p. 115.
12. Ibid.
13. Bader, 1969.
14. Tarassov, 1971.
15. Duarte et al., 1999.
16. Formicola and Buzhilova, 2004.

17. Harrold, 1980.
18. Larsson, 1983.
19. Albrethsen and Petersen, 1976.
20. Janik, 2000.
21. Thomas, et al., 2011.
22. Finlay, 2000.
23. Cooney, 1992.
24. Finlay, 2000, p. 418.
25. Ibid.
26. Ibid.
27. Boric and Stefanovic, 2004, p. 540.
28. Ibid.
29. This argument is somewhat faulty as the remains could not be sexed and grave goods are not necessarily indicative of gender or age, per Scott, 1999.
30. Scott, 1999.
31. Moses, 2008.
32. Moses, 2008.
33. Ibid.
34. Orrelle, 2008.
35. Ibid.
36. Artin, 2008.
37. Moses, 2008.
38. Le Mort, 2008.
39. Lillie, 2008, p. 33.
40. Pomadère, 2008.
41. Scott, 1999.
42. Andreeva, 2008.
43. Dervin, 2010.
44. Ibid.
45. Gamble, 2008.
46. Knight, 2008, p. 76.
47. Scott, 1999.
48. Ibid.

Chapter 3

1. Colon and Colon, 2001.
2. Ibid.
3. Diodorus Siculus, quoted in Colon and Colon, 2001.
4. Colon and Colon, 2001.

5. Ibid.
6. Ibid.
7. Kalish, 1980.
8. Mizoguchi, 2000.
9. Donnelly and Murphy, 2008.
10. Rawson, 2003.
11. Tsaliki, 2008.
12. Taylor, 2008.
13. Rawson, 2003.
14. Jesch, 1991, p. 118.
15. From the Oxyrhynchus Papyri 744, cited in Colon and Colon, 2001.
16. Scott, 1999.
17. Ibid.
18. Charlier, 2008.
19. Sirbu, 2008.
20. Ibid.
21. Scott, 1999.
22. Golden, 1988, p. 156.
23. Binford, 1972.
24. Cicero, 2002.
25. Houby-Nielsen, 2000.
26. Ibid.
27. Crawford, 2000.
28. Ibid.
29. Ibid.
30. Payne, 1916, p. 170.
31. Stager et al, 1984.
32. Plutarch, 1927; Colon and Colon, 2001.
33. deMause, 1974, p. 28.
34. Payne, 1916.
35. Feitosa, 2010.
36. Colon and Colon, 2001.
37. Kinney, 2004, p. 170–171.
38. Hsu and Ward, 1984.
39. Kinney, 2004, p. 83.
40. Payne, 1916.
41. Ibid.
42. Colon and Colon, 2001.
43. Vreeland and Cockburn, 1980.
44. Ibid.
45. Colon and Colon, 2001.

46. Kalish, 1980.
47. Colon and Colon, 2001.
48. Feitosa et al., 2010.
49. Colon and Colon, 2001.
50. Du Chaillu, 1889.
51. Du Chaillu, 1889.
52. Fischer, 1980.

Chapter 4

1. Wilson, 1984.
2. Herlihy, 1997.
3. Ibid.
4. Ibid.
5. Colon and Colon, 2001.
6. Ibid.
7. Quoted in Groenendijk, van Lieburg, and Exalto, 2010, p. 275.
8. Ibid, p. 285.
9. Ibid, p. 283.
10. Colon and Colon, 2001.
11. Ibid.
12. Ibid.
13. King, 1991, p. 9–10.
14. Shahar, 1990.
15. Kinney, 2004, p. 171.
16. Kinney, 2004, p. 172.
17. Colon and Colon, 2001.
18. Billings, 1987.
19. Colon and Colon, 2001.
20. Gil'adi, 1993; deMause, 1974.
21. Ibid.
22. Ibid., p. 378.
23. Aries, 1981.
24. Murpy, 2011.
25. Donnelly and Murphy, 2008.
26. Hannawalt, 1995.
27. Ibid.
28. Finlay, 2000, p. 413.
29. Murphy, 2011.
30. Ibid.

31. Ibid.
32. King, 1994.
33. Labno, 2011, p. 150; Langmuir, 2006.
34. Labno, 2011, p. 200.
35. Labno, 2011.
36. Weiss-Krejci, 2008.

Chapter 5

1. Burns, 1990.
2. Dye and Smith, 1986.
3. Ibid., p. 337.
4. Dye and Smith, 1986, p. 330.
5. Ibid.
6. Florence Kelley, quoted in Dye and Smith, 1986.
7. Dye and Smith, 1986.
8. Pollock, 1983.
9. McMahon, 2012, p. 46.
10. Dye and Smith, 1986, p. 334, from "The Diary of Mary (Vial) Holyoke, 1760–1800).
11. Smart, 1993 p. 52.
12. Smart, 1993.
13. Dye and Smith, 1986, p. 335.
14. Smart, 1993.
15. Ibid.
16. Davis, 2009.
17. Vovelle, 1980, p. 540.
18. Ibid, p. 543.
19. Slater, 1977.
20. Schlissel, 1982.
21. Teelucksingh, 2006.
22. Ibid. Teelucksingh, 2006 notes that a planter in Sheridan's *Doctors and Slaves*, discusses the efforts of slave girls in British West India to preserve themselves through abortions.
23. Savitt, 1975; Kiple and Kiple, 1977.
24. Ibid.
25. Ibid.
26. Ucko, 1969.
27. Jamieson, 1995.
28. DiGirolamo, 2002.
29. Ibid.

30. Taylor, 1983.
31. DiGirolamo, 2002, p. 22.
32. DiGirolamo, 2002.
33. Ibid., p. 25.
34. Taylor, 1983.
35. Landis, 1896.
36. Sambrook, 1999.
37. Ibid.
38. Ibid.
39. Clayton, 2009.
40. Caron, 2010.
41. Burnston, 1982.

Chapter 6

1. CDC, 2010.
2. Kübler-Ross, 1983.
3. Smart, 1993.
4. Kübler-Ross, 1983.
5. Suzuki, 2003.
6. Kübler-Ross, 1983, p. 129.
7. Ibid.
8. Ibid.
9. Jones, 1988.
10. Ibid.
11. Levine, 1997.
12. Dignity Memorial, 2014.
13. Scott, 1999.
14. Murphy, 2011, quotes Christine Moulder, 1998 with respect to parental grief over stillbirth.
15. Reid, 2013.
16. Morgan, 2009.
17. CNN, 2014.
18. Nuwer, 2014.
19. Smith-Spark and Magnay, 2014.
20. Parent and Shevell, 1998.
21. Scheper-Hughes, 1989.
22. Ibid.
23. Ibid.
24. Scheper-Hughes, 1989, p. 189.

25. Nations, 2013.
26. BenEzer, 2004.
27. Nations, 2013, p. 677.
28. Ibid., p. 669.
29. Ibid, p. 663.
30. Kalish, 1980.
31. Filler, 2012.
32. Ibid.
33. Shultz et al., 2013.
34. Schaller and Nightingale, 1992.
35. CDC, 2010.
36. Eisenberg, 1982, p. xvi.
37. Volavkova, 1994, p. 39.

Chapter 7

1. World Bank, 2014.
2. Newell, 2008.
3. Ibid.
4. Opler and Bittle, 1961.
5. El-Najjar and Mulinski, 1980.
6. Ibid.
7. Darlington, 1930.
8. Taylor, 1983.
9. Darlington, 1930.
10. Feitosa et al., 2010, pp. 854–855.
11. Feitosa et al., 2010.
12. Ibid.
13. de Azara, 1809.
14. Dervin, 2010.
15. Harris, 1982.
16. Kalish, 1980.
17. Murray, 1912.
18. Hausfater and Hrdy, 2008.
19. Williamson, 1978.
20. Scott, 1999.
21. Colon and Colon, 2001.
22. Ibid.
23. Ibid.
24. Williamson, 1978.

25. Colon and Colon, 2001.
26. Ibid.
27. Boric and Stefanovic, 2004.
28. Bendann, 1930, p. 204.
29. Hertz, 1960.
30. Darlington, 1930.
31. Pretty and Calder, 1980.
32. Rosenblatt, 1997.
33. Nations, 2013.

Chapter 8

1. Babu, Oct. 23, 2011.
2. Smith, 1985.
3. Baun, 1994.
4. Colon, 2001 p. 502.
5. Hanawalt, 1993.
6. Herlihy, 1997.
7. Burns, 2011.
8. Smith, 1985.
9. Ibid., p. 546.
10. Ibid.
11. Colon and Colon, 2001.
12. Feitosa, 2010, p. 860.
13. Ibid.
14. Oneworldnews.org.
15. Chrisman, 1920.
16. Doyle, 2008.
17. Doyle, 2008, p. 373.
18. Ibid., p. 375.
19. Doyle, 2008.
20. Suzman, 1994, p. 259.
21. Knodel, 1982.
22. Palloni and Rafalimanana, 1999.
23. Grieser et al., 2001.
24. Poznanski, 1972.
25. Ibid.

Chapter 9

1. Duhl, 1999.
2. Baltussen, 2009.
3. Ibid., p. 8.
4. Carroll, 2006, p. 611.
5. Dorandi, 1999.
6. Cicero, 2002.
7. Rawson, 2003 p. 282.
8. Gil'adi, 1992.
9. Gil'adi, 1993.
10. Gil'adi, 1989.
11. Ibid.
12. Ibid.
13. Gil'adi, 1989, p. 43.
14. Gil'adi, 1993, p. 368.
15. Ibid., p. 373.
16. Kochanowski, 1995.
17. Kochanowski, 2008.
18. Linton, 2008, p. 3.
19. Ibid.
20. Linton, 2008, p. 29.
21. Duhl, 1999.
22. Kramer, 1998.
23. Kramer, 1998, p. 34.
24. Kliger in Kramer, 1998, p. 38, "The Last Cradle Song".
25. Lerner, 1997, p. 41.
26. Ibid., p. 42.
27. McMahon, 2012, p. 28; p. 32, p. 37.
28. McMahon, 2012, p. 40.
29. Douglas, 1977 quoted in Simonds and Katz Rothman, 1992, p. 6.
30. Simonds and Katz Rothman, 1992.
31. Ibid., p. 102–3.
32. Ibid., p. 101.
33. Crooker, 1984 in Simonds and Roth Kathman, 1992.
34. Skeath, in Simonds and Roth Kathman, 1992, p. 250.

Chapter 10

1. Schaller, 2001.
2. Beattie, 2006.
3. Van Setten, 1999.
4. Langmuir, 2006, p. 69.
5. Huskinson, 2005.
6. Langmuir, 2006, p. 75.
7. Ibid.
8. Burns, 2002.
9. Burns, 1990.
10. Burns, 2002.
11. Burns, 1990.
12. Burns, 2002, image 9.
13. Burns, 1990, image 18.
14. Van Setten, 1999.
15. Schaller, 2001.
16. Van Setten, 1999.
17. Ibid.
18. Burns, 2011.

Chapter 11

1. Williamson, 1978, p. 61.
2. Scott, 1999.
3. Ibid.
4. Scott, 1999.
5. Piers, 1978.
6. Ibid.
7. Scott, 1999.
8. Piers, 1978.
9. Ibid.
10. Hoffer and Hull, 1981.
11. Scott, 1999.
12. Hoffer and Hull, 1981.
13. Ibid.
14. Birdsell, 1986, p. 239.
15. Divale, 1972.
16. Mays, 1993.
17. Boswell, 1984.

18. Bowen, 2002; Lammens 1987.
19. Smith, 1903.
20. Shiono, et al., 1986.
21. Payne, 1916.
22. Westermarck, 1968.
23. AFP, 2011.
24. deMause, 1974.
25. Scott, 1999, p. 82.
26. Scott, 1999.
27. Ibid.
28. Scott, 1999, p. 86.
29. Payne, 1916.
30. Golden, 1988.

References

AFP. January 18, 2011. Infanticide on the rise: 1,210 babies found dead in 2010, says Edhi. *The Tribune.*

Albrethsen, S.E. and Petersen, E.B. 1976. Excavation of a Mesolithic cemetery at Vaedbek, Denmark. *Acta Archaeologica* 47: 3–28.

Alexiou, Margaret. 1974. *The ritual lament in Greek tradition.* London: Cambridge University Press.

Ali, Mohamed M., Blacker, John, and Gareth Jones. 2003. Annual mortality rates and excess deaths of children under five in Iraq, 1991–98. *Population Studies* 57(2): 217–226.

Allen, Nicholas, Callan, Hilary, Dunbar, Robin, and Wendy James. 2011. *Early human kinship: From sex to social reproduction.* Massachusetts: Blackwell Publishing.

Andreeva, Marina. 2008. Pre-adult and adult burials of East Manych catacomb culture: Was infanticide really impossible. In *Babies reborn*, ed. K. Bŭchvarov, 149–160. Oxford: Archaeopress.

Aries, Philippe, 1973. *Centuries of childhood: A social history of family life.* Translated by Robert Baldick. London: Harmondsworth.

Aries, Philippe. 1981. *The hour of our death: The classic history of western attitudes toward death over the last one thousand years.* New York: Vintage Books.

Artin, Gassia. 2008. The jar burials of the Chalcolithic "Necropolis" at Byblos. In *Babies reborn*, ed. K. Bŭchvarov, 79–86. Oxford: Archaeopress.

Babu, Chaya. October 23, 2011. *Indian girls shed 'unwanted' names.* Associated Press.

Bader, Otto. 1978. *Sungir Upper Paleolithic site.* Moscow: Nauka.

Baltussen, Han. 2009. Personal grief and public mourning in Plutarch's consolation to his wife. *American Journal of Philology* 130(1): 67–98.

Baun, Jane. 1994. The fate of babies dying before baptism in Byzantium. In *The Church and Childhood,* ed. D. Wood, 117–118. Oxford: Blackwells.

Beattie, Kathryn. 2006. *Aspects of acceptance and denial in painted posthumous portraits and post-mortem photographs of nineteenth-century children.* Unpublished Master's Thesis: Concordia University, Canada.

Bendann, Effie. 1930. *Death customs: An analytic study of burial rites.* New York: Alfred A. Knopf.

BenEzer, G. 2004. Trauma signals in life. In *Trauma: Life stories of survivors,* eds. K. Rogers, S. Leydesdorff, and G. Dawson, 29–42. New Brunswick: Transaction Publishers.

Billings, Malcolm. 1988. *The cross and the crescent: A History of the crusades.* Sterling Publishing Company.

Binford, Lewis Robert. 1972. *An archaeological perspective.* London: Academic Press.

Birdsell, Joseph, B. 1986. Some predictions for the Pleistocene based on equilibrium systems among recent hunter gatherers. In *Man the hunter*, eds. Richard Lee & Irven DeVore, 229–249. Chicago: Aldine Publishing.

Bloch, Maurice, and Jonathan Parry. 1982. *Death and the regeneration of life.* Cambridge University Press.

Boric, Dusan and S. Stefanovic. 2004. Birth and death: Infant burials from Vlasac and Lepenski Vir. *Antiquity* 78(301): 526–546.

Boswell, John Eastburn. 1984. Exposition and oblation: the abandonment of children and the ancient and medieval family. *American Historical Review* 8(1): 10–33.

Bowen, Donna Lee. 2002. "Infanticide," in *Encyclopedia of the Qur'an.*

Breschi, Marco, Lucia Pozzi, and Società italiana di demografia storica. 2004. *The determinants of infant and child mortality in past European populations.* Udine: Forum Press.

Bŭchvarov, Krum, and International Union of Prehistoric and Protohistoric Sciences. 2008. *Babies reborn: Infant/child burials in Pre- and Protohistory.* Oxford: Archaeopress.

Burns, Stanley B. 1990. *Sleeping beauty: Memorial photography in America.* Santa Fe: Twelvetress Press.

Burns, Stanley B. 2002. *Sleeping beauty II: Grief, bereavement and the family memorial photography, American and European traditions.* New York: Burns Archive Press.

Burns, Stanley B. 2011. *Sleep beauty III: Memorial photography, the children.* New York: Burns Archive Press.

Burnston, Sharon Ann. 1982. Babies in the well: An underground insight into deviant behavior in eighteenth-century Philadelphia. *The Pennsylvania Magazine of History and Biography* 106(2): 151–186.

Caron, Simone. 2010. 'Killed by its mother': Infanticide in Providence County, Rhode Island, 1870–1938. *Journal of Social History* 44(1): 213–237.

Carroll, M. 2006. *Spirits of the dead: Roman funerary commemoration in Western art.* Oxford. New York: Oxford University Press.

Center for Disease Control and Prevention. 2010. Ten leading causes of death and injury—PDFs|Injury Center|CDC."

Center for Disease Control and Prevention. 2011. CDC Features—CDC Analysis supports declaration of famine and humanitarian disaster in Somalia. http://www.cdc.gov/Features/Africa Famine/

Charlier, Philippe. 2008. The value of paleoteratology and forensic pathology for the understanding of atypical burials: Two Mediterranean examples from the field. In *Deviant burial* ed. E. M. Murphy, 57–70. Oxford: Oxbow Books.

Chrisman, O. 1920. *The historical child.* Boston: Richard G. Badger.

CIA. 2014. *World Fact Book.* https://www.cia.gov/library/publications/the-world-factbook/rankorder/2223rank.html

Cicero, Marcus Tullius. 2002. *Cicero on the emotions: Tusculan disputations 3 and 4.* Chicago: University of Chicago Press.

Clayton, Mary. 2009. Changes in Old Bailey trials for the murder of newborn babies, 1674–1803, *Continuity and Change* 24(2): 337–359.

Cockburn, Aidan, Eve Cockburn, and Theodore A. Reyman. 1980. *Mummies, disease and ancient cultures.* Cambridge University Press.

Colon, A.R., and Colon, P.A. 2001. *A history of children: A socio-cultural survey across millennia.* Westport, Connecticut: Greenwood Press.

Cooney, Gabriel. 1992. Body politics and grave messages: Irish Neolithic mortuary practices. In *Vessels for the Ancestors,* eds. A. Sheridan and N. Sharples, 128–142. Edinburgh: Edinburgh University Press.

Crawford, Sally. 2000. Children, Grave Goods and Social Status in Early Anglo-Saxon England. In *Children and material culture,* ed. J.S. Derevenski, 169–179. Florence, Kentucky: Routledge.

Darlington, H. S. 1930. Ceremonial behaviorism. *Psychoanalytic Review* 18: 180–328.

Davis, Gayle. 2009. Stillbirth registration and perceptions of infant death, 1900–60: the Scottish case in national context. *The Economic History Review* 62(3): 629–654.

de Azara, Felix. 1809. *Voyages dans l'Amerique Meridionale, vol .2.*

deMause, Lloyd. 1974. *The history of childhood.* New York: Psychohistory Press.

Derevenski, Joanna Sofaer. 1994. Where are the children? Accessing children in the past. *Archaeological Review from Cambridge* 13(2): 7–20.

Derevenski, Joanna Sofaer. 2000. *Children and material culture.* Florence, Kentucky: Routledge.

Derosas, Renzo. 2003. Watch out for the children! Differential infant mortality of jews and catholics in nineteenth-century Venice. *Historical Methods: A Journal of Quantitative and Interdisciplinary History* 36 (3): 109–30.

Dervin, Dan. 2010. The prehistory of parenting and the enigma of fire. *The Journal of Psychohistory* 37(4): 349–365.

DiGirolamo, Vincent. 2002. Newsboy funerals: Tales of sorrow and solidarity in urban America. *Journal of Social History* 36(1): 5–30.

DignityMemorial.com. *Prayer at the grave of a child.* http://www.dignitymemorial.com/en-us/library/article/name/scripture-prayer-at-the-grave-of-a-child

Divale, William T. 1972. Systemic population control in the middle and upper Palaeolithic: Inferences based on contemporary hunter-gatherers. *World Archaeology* 4(2): 222–43.

Donnelly, Colm J. and Murphy, Eileen M. 2008. The origins of *cillini* in Ireland. In *Deviant burial* ed. E. M. Murphy, 191–223. Oxford: Oxbow Books.

Dorandi, Tiziano. 1999. Chapter 2: Chronology. In *The Cambridge history of Hellenistic,* ed. Algra et al., 8. Cambridge.

Doyle, Shawn. 2008. The child of death: Personal names and parental attitudes toward mortality in Bunyoro, Western Uganda, 1900–2005. *Journal of African History* 49: 361–382.

Duarte C, Maurı'cio J, Pettitt P.B., Souto P., Trinkaus E. and van der Plicht H, Zilha˜o J. 1999. The early Upper Paleolithic human skeleton from the Abrigo do Lagar Velho (Portugal) and modern human emergence in Iberia. *Proceedings of the National Academy of the Sciences USA* 96:7604–7609.

Du Chaillu, Paul B. 1889. *The Viking age.* New York: Scribner.

Duhl, Lisa S. 1999. *Rocking an empty cradle: A psychological study of Yiddish Holocaust lullabies.* Unpublished Dissertation, California School of Psychology, Berkeley, CA.

Dye, Nancy Schrom and Smith, Daniel Blake. 1986. Mother love and infant death, 1750–1920. *Journal of American History* 73(2): 329–353.

Edvinsson, S. (2004). Social Differences in Infant and Child Mortality in Nineteenth Century Sweden. In *The determinants of infant and child,* eds. M. Breschi, L. Pozzi. Udine: Forum Press.

Eisenberg, Azriel Louis. 1982. *The lost generation: Children in the Holocaust.* New York: Pilgrim Press.

El-Najjar, Mahmoud Y. and Thomas M. Mulinski. 1980. Mummies and mummification practices in the Southwestern and Southern United States. In *Mummies, disease,* eds. A. Cockburn, E. Cockburn, and T.A. Reyman, 103–177. Cambridge University Press.

Feitosa, Saulo Ferreira, Volnei Garrafa, Gabriele Cornelli, Carla Tardivo, and Samuel José de Carvalho. 2010. Bioethics, culture andiInfanticide in Brazilian indigenous communities: The Zuruahá case. *Cadernos de Saúde Pública* 26(5): 853–65.

Fildes, V. 1986. *Breasts, bottles, and babies.* Edinburg: Edinburgh University Press.

Filler, Lane. 2014. Why the Sandy Hook Elementary School shooting feels different—Lane Filler. *Newsday.* http://www.newsday.com/opinion/columnists/lane-filler/filler-why-the-sandy-hook-elementary-school-shooting-feels-different-1.4334509

Finlay, Nyree. 2000. Outside of life: Traditions of infant burial in Ireland from *cillin* to cist. *World Archaeology* 31(3): 407–422.

Fischer, Christian. 1980. Bog bodies of Denmark. In *Mummies, disease,* eds. A. Cockburn, E. Cockburn, and T.A. Reyman, 177–193. Cambridge University Press.

Formicola, Vincenzo and Buzhilova, Alexandra P. 2004. Double child burial from Sunghir (Russia): Pathology and inferences for Upper Paleolithic funerary practices. *American Journal of Physical Anthropology* 124: 189–198.

Gamble, Clive. 2008. Kinship and material culture: Archaeological implications of the human global diaspora. In *Kinship and Evolution,* eds. J. Allen, H. Callan, R. Dunbar, and W. James, 27–40. Oxford: Blackwell.

Gil'adi, Avner. 1989. Sabr (steadfastness) of bereaved parents: A motif in medieval Muslim consolation treatises and some parallels in Jewish writings. *The Jewish Quarterly Review* 80(1/2): 35–48.

Gil'adi, Avner. 1992. *Children of Islam: Concepts of childhood in medieval Muslim society.* New York: St. Martin's Press.

Gil'adi, Avner. 1993. The child was small…Not so the grief for him: Sources, structure, and content of Al-Sakhawi's consolation treatise for bereaved parents. *Poetics Today* 14(2): 367–386.

Goldberg, Susan. 1977. Infant development and mother-infant interaction in urban Zambia, In *Culture and infancy,* eds. Leiderman, P.H., Tulkin, S.R. and A. Rosenfeld, 211–244. New York: Academic Press, Inc.

Golden, Mark. 1988. Did the ancients care when their children died. *Greece & Rome* 35(2): 152–163.

Grieser, Mira, Joel Gittelsohn, Anita V. Shankar, Todd Koppenhaver, Thomas K. Legrand, Ravai Marindo, Webster M. Mavhu, and Kenneth Hill. 2001. Reproductive decision making and the HIV/AIDS epidemic in Zimbabwe. *Journal of Southern African Studies* 27 (2): 225–43.

Groenendijk, Leendert F., Fred A. van Lieburg, and John Exalto. 2010. Away with all my pleasant things in the world…': Model death-bed accounts of two young victims of the plague of 1664 in the Dutch town of Leyden. *Paedagogica Historica* 46 (3): 271–288.

Guha-Sapir, Debarati, and Willem Gijsbert Panhuis. 2004. Conflict-related mortality: An analysis of 37 datasets." *Disasters* 28 (4): 418–428.

Hanawalt, Barbara A. 1993. *Growing up in medieval London: The experience of childhood in history.* New York: Oxford University Press.

Harris, Olivia. 1982. The dead and the devils among the Bolivian Laymi. In Death and the regeneration, eds. M. Bloch, and J. Parry, 45. Cambridge University Press.

Harrold, F. 1980. A comparative analysis of Eurasian Palaeolithic burials. *World Archaeology* 12(2): 195–211.

Hausfater, Glenn, and Sarah Blaffer Hrdy. 2008. *Infanticide: Comparative and Evolutionary Perspectives.* Transaction Publishers.

Herlihy, Davidson. 1997. *The Black Death and the transformation of the West.* Cambridge: Harvard University Press.

Hertz, R. 1960. *Death and the Right Hand.* Translated by Rodney and Claudia Needham. Illinois: Glencoe.

Hoffer, Peter Charles, and N. E. H Hull. 1981. *Murdering mothers: Infanticide in England and New England, 1558–1803.* New York: New York University Press.

Houby-Nielsen, Sanne. 2000. Child Burials in Ancient Athens. In *Children and material culture,* ed. J.S. Derevenski, 151–166. Florence, Kentucky: Routledge.

Hsu, C.H. and A.H. Ward. 1984. *Ancient Chinese society.* San Francisco: Yee Wen Publishing.

Huskinson, Janet. 2005. Disappearing children? Children in Roman funerary art of the first to the fourth century AD. In *Hoping for continuity,* eds. K. Mustakallio, J. Hanska, H. Sainio and V. Vuolanto, 91–103. Rome: Acta Instituti Romani Finlandiae.

Iwaniec, Dorota. 2004. *Children who fail to thrive: A practice guide.* Hoboken: John Wiley & Sons.

Jamieson, R.W. 1995. Material culture and social death: African-American burial practices. *Historical Archaeology*: 39–58.

Janik, Liliana. 2000. The construction of individual among Northern European fisher-gatherhunters in the early and mid-Pleistocene. In *Children and material culture,* ed. J.S. Derevenski, 117–130. Florence, Kentucky: Routledge.

Jesch, Judith. 1991. *Women in the Viking Age.* Boydell & Brewer Ltd.

Jones, H. Julie. 1988. The importance of children's funerals in the mourning process. *Bereavement Care,* 7(3): 34–37.

Jordon, T.E. 1987. *Victorian childhood.* Albany: State University of New York Press.

Kalish, Richard A. 1980. *Death and dying: Views from many cultures.* Baywood Publishing.

Kent, George. 1991. *The politics of children's survival.* New York: Praeger.

King, Margaret L. 1991. *Women of the Renaissance.* Chicago: University of Chicago Press.

King, Margaret L. 1994. *The death of the child Valerio Marcello.* Chicago: University of Chicago Press.

Kinney, A. B. 2004. *Representations of childhood and youth in early China.* California: Stanford University Press.

Kiple, K.F., and V.H. Kiple. 1977. Slave child mortality: Some nutritional answers to a perennial puzzle. *Journal of Social History* 10(3): 284–309.

Knight, Chris. 2008. Early human kinship was matrilineal. In *Kinship and Evolution*, eds. J. Allen, H. Callan, R. Dunbar, and W. James, 61–82. Oxford: Blackwell.

Knodel, J. 1982. Child mortality and reproductive behaviour in German village populations in the past: A micro-level analysis of the replacement effect. *Population Studies* 36(2): 177–200.

Kochanowski, Jan. 1995. *Laments.* Translated by Stanisław Barańczak and Seamus Heaney, New York: Farrar, Strauss and Giroux.

Kochanowski, Jan. 2008. *Laments.* Translated by Dorothea Prall. http://www.gutenberg.org/ebooks/27179

Kohl, Marvin. 1978. *Infanticide and the value of life.* Buffalo, N.Y.: Prometheus Books.

Kramer, Aaron. 1998. *The Last Lullaby: Poetry from the Holocaust.* New York: Syracuse University Press.

Kübler-Ross, Elisabeth. 1983. *On children and death.* Touchstone: New York.

Kurtz, Donna C. and Boardman, John. 1971. *Greek burial customs.* Ithaca: Cornell University Press.

Labno, Jeannie. 2011. *Commemorating the Polish Renaissance child: Funeral monuments and their European context.* Burlington: Ashgate Publishing Company.

Lammens, Henri. 1987. *Islam: Belief and institutions.* London: Methuen & Co. Ltd.

Landis, E. B. 1896. Mourning and Burial Rites of Korea. *Journal of the Anthropological Institute of Great Britain and Ireland*: 340–61.

Langmuir, Erika. 2006. *Imagining childhood.* Yale University Press: London Larsson, Lars. 1983. The Skateholm project: A late Mesolithic settlement and cemetery Complex at a southern Swedish bay. *Meddelanden fran Lunds Universitets Historiska Museum* (5)19: 5–38.

Le Mort, Françoise. 2008. Infant burials in Pre-Pottery Neolithic Cyprus: Evidence from Khirokitia. In *Babies reborn*, ed. K. Bŭchvarov, 23–32. Oxford: Archaeopress.

Lerner, Laurence.1997. *Angels and Absences: Child Deaths in the Nineteenth Century.* London: Vanderbilt University Press.

Levine, E. 1997. Jewish views and customs on death. In *Death and bereavement,* eds. C.M. Parkes, P. Laungani, and B. Young, 98–130. London: Routledge.

Lillie, Malcolm. 2008. Suffer the children: 'Visualising' children in the archaeological record. Infant burials in Pre-Pottery Neolithic Cyprus. In *Babies reborn*, ed. K. Bŭchvarov, 33–44. Oxford: Archaeopress.

Linton, Anna. 2008. *Poetry and Parental Bereavement in Early Modern Lutheran Germany.* New York: Oxford University Press.

Mays, Simon 1993. Infanticide in Roman Britain. *Antiquity* 67: 883–888.

McMahon, Lucia. 2012. 'So truly afflicting and distressing to me his sorrowing mother': Expressions of maternal grief in eighteenth-century Philadelphia. *Journal of the Early Republic* 32(1): 27–60.

Mizoguchi, Koji. 2000. The child as node of past, present and future. In *Children and material culture,* ed. J.S. Derevenski, 141–150. Florence, Kentucky: Routledge.

Morgan, Darla. 2009. Caring for dying children: Assessing the needs of the pediatric palliative care nurse. *Pediatric Nursing* 35(2): 86–90.

Moses, Sharon. 2008. Catalhöyük's foundation burials: Ritual child sacrifice or convenient deaths? In *Babies reborn,* ed. K. Bŭchvarov, 45–52. Oxford: Archaeopress.

Moulder, C. 1998. *Understanding pregnancy loss.* London: Macmillan.

Munro, Robin, and Human Rights Watch/Asia. 1996. *Death by default: A policy of fatal neglect in China's state orphanages.* Human Rights Watch. http://www.hrw.org/reports/1996/01/01/death-default

Murphy, Eileen M. 2008. *Deviant burial in the archaeological record.* Oxford: Oxbow Books.

Murphy, Eileen M. 2011. Children's burial grounds in Ireland (Cillini) and parental emotions toward infant death. *International Journal of Historical Archaeology* 15(3): 409–28.

Murray, J. H. P. 1912. *Papua or British New Guinea.* London: T. Fisher Undwin.

Mustakallio, Katariina, Hanska, Jussi, Sainio, Hanna-Leena, and Vuolanto, Ville. 2005. *Hoping for continuity: Childhood, education and death in Antiquity and the Middle Ages.* Rome: Acta Instituti Romani Finlandiae.

Nations, Marilyn. 2013. Dead-baby dreams, transfiguration and recovery from infant death trauma in Northeast Brazil. *Transcultural Psychiatry* 50: 662–882.

Newell, Quincy D. 2008. The varieties of religious experience: Baptized Indians at Mission San Francisco de Asís, 1776–1821. *The American Indian Quarterly* 32(4): 412–42.

Nuwer, Rachel. 2014. The world needs to talk about child euthanasia. *New Scientist.* http://www.hrw.org/reports/1996/01/01/death-default

Oneworldnews.org. 1995. The dying rooms special report. http://www.taliacarner.com/thedyingroomsspecialreport.html

Opler, Morris E., and William E. Bittle. 1961. The death practices and eschatology of the Kiowa Apache. *Southwestern Journal of Anthropology*: 383–94.

Oris, Michael, Neven, Muriel, and Alter, George. 2004. Maternal depletion and the survival chances of infants and children in nineteenth-century Eastern Belgium. In *The determinants of infant and child,* eds. M. Breschi, L. Pozzi, 153–173. Udine: Forum Press.

Orrelle, Estelle. 2008. Infant jar burials-a ritual associated with early agriculture? In *Babies reborn,* ed. K. Bŭchvarov, 71–78. Oxford: Archaeopress.

Palloni, Alberto, and Hantamala Rafalimanana. 1999. The effects of infant mortality on fertility revisited: New evidence from Latin America. *Demography* 36(1): 41–58.

Parent, Stefan and Shevell, Michael. 1998. The "first to perish": Child euthanasia in the Third Reich. *Archives of Pediatric Adolescent Medicine* 152: 79–86.

Parkes, Collin Murray, Laungani, Pittu, and Young, Bill. 1997. *Death and bereavement across cultures.* London: Routledge.

Payne, George Henry. 1916. *The child in human progress.* New York: G.P. Putnam's Sons.

Plutarch. 1927. *Moralia.* Translated by F.C. Babbitt. London: William Heinemann.

Pollock, Linda, A. 1983. *Forgotten children: Parent-child relations from 1500 to 1900.* New York: Cambridge University.

Pomadère, Maia. 2008. Des morts peu fiables: Les sépultures néolithiques d'immatures en Gréce. In *Babies reborn*, ed. K. Bŭchvarov, 53–60. Oxford: Archaeopress.

Potter, Ben A., Irish, Joel D., Reuther, Joshua D., Gelvin-Reymiller, Carol., and Holliday, Vance T. 2011. A Terminal Pleistocene child cremation and residential structure from Eastern Beringia. *Science* 331(6020): 1058–1062.

Poznanski, Elva Orlow 1972. "The 'replacement child': A saga of unresolved parental grief." *The Journal of Pediatrics* 81 (6): 1190–93.

Preston, Samuel H. and Haines, Michael R. 1991. *Fatal years: Child mortality in late nineteenth-century America.* New Jersey: Princeton University Press.

Pretty, Graeme L. and Angela Calder. 1980. Mummification in Australia and Melanesia. In *Mummies, disease,* eds. A. Cockburn, E. Cockburn, and T.A. Reyman, 289–307. Cambridge University Press.

Raczek, Teresa. 2003. Subsistence strategies and burial rituals: Social practices in the Late Deccan Chalcolithic. *Asian Perspectives* 42 (2): 247–66.

Rawson, Beryl. 2003. Death, burial, and commemoration of children in Roman Italy. In *Early Christian Families,* Eds. D. L. Balch and C. Osiek, Carolyn, 277–297. Grand Rapids: William B. Eerdsman Publishing Company.

Razzel, Peter and Christine Spence. 2004. Poverty or disease environment? The history of mortality in Britain 1500–1950. In *The determinants of infant and child,* eds. M. Breschi, L. Pozzi, 43–65. Udine: Forum Press.

Reher, David S., and Alberto Sanz Gimeno. 2004. Childhood mortality patterns in Spain before and during the demographic transition: In search of new dimensions. In *The determinants of infant and child,* eds. M. Breschi, L. Pozzi, 19–42. Udine: Forum Press.

Reid, Alice, Davies, Ros, Garrett, Eilidh, and Blaikie, Andrew. 2006. Vulnerability among illegitimate children in nineteenth century Scotland. *Annales de Demographie Historique,* 1: 89–113.

Reid, Fiona. 2013. Grief and the experiences of nurses providing palliative care to children and young people at home. *Nursing Children and Young People* 25 (9): 31–36.

Rosenblatt, P.C. 1997. Grief in small-scale societies. In *Death and bereavement,* eds. C.M. Parkes, P. Laungani, and B. Young, 27–51. London: Routledge.

Roveland, Blythe. 2008. Footprints in the clay: Upper Palaeolithic children in ritual and secular contexts. In *Children and material culture,* ed. J.S. Derevenski, 29–36. Florence, Kentucky: Routledge.

Russell, Beth. 2007. The mystery of China's orphans. *The New York Times.* http://www.nytimes.com/2007/02/01/opinion/01iht-edrussell.html

Saha, Unnati Rani and van Soest, Arthur. 2011. Infant death clustering in families: Magnitude, causes, and the influence of better health services, Bangladesh 1982–2005. *Population Studies* 65(3): 273–287.

Sambrook, Pamela A. 1999. Unfair and unprotected: Community responses to the sudden deaths of children in Staffordshire in 1851 and 1860. *Family & Community History* 2(2): 85–99.

Savitt, Todd L. 1975. Smothering and overlaying of Virginia slave children: A suggested explanation. *Bulletin of the History of Medicine* 49(3): 400–404.

Schaller, Jane Green and Nightingale, Elena O. 1992. Children and childhoods: Hidden casualties of war and civil unrest. *JAMA* 269(5): 642–644.

Schaller, Wendy McPeters. 2001. *Children borne aloft: Nicolaes Maes's Ganymede portraiture and the context of death and mourning in the seventeenth-century Netherlands.* Unpublished Dissertation, Ohio State University, Ohio.

Scheper-Hughes, Nancy. 1989. Death without weeping: Has poverty ravaged mother love in the shanty towns of Brazil? *Natural History* 98(10): 8–16.

Scheper-Hughes, Nancy. 1992. *Death without weeping: The violence of everyday life in Brazil.* Berkeley: University of California Press.

Schlissel, L. 1982. *Women's diaries of the Westward journey.* New York: Schocken Books.

Schmelz, U.O. 1971. *Infant and early childhood mortality among the Jews of the diaspora.* Jerusalem, Institute of Contemporary Jewry, Hebrew University.

Schultz, James. A. 1995. *The knowledge of childhood in the German Middle Ages, 1100–1350.* University of Pennsylvania Press.

Scott, Eleanor. 1999. *The archaeology of infancy and infant death.* Oxford: BAR International.

Shahar, Shulasmith. 1990. *Childhood in the Middle Ages.* New York: Routledge.

Shultz, James M., Muschert, Glenn W., Dingwall, Alison, Cohen, Alyssa M., Loayza-Alarico, Manuel J., Lescano, Andres G., Suarez-Ognio, Luis A., Ramirez-Prada, Gladys M., Blazes, David L. and Xiaodong Sun. 2013. The Sandy Hook elementary school Shooting as tipping point: 'This time is different.' *Disaster Health.* 1(2). http://www.landesbioscience.com/journals/disasterhealth/2012dh001r.pdf

Shiono, Hiroshi; Atoyo Maya, Noriko Tabata, Masataka Fujiwara, Jun-ich Azumi and Mashahiko Morita. 1986. Medicolegal aspects of infanticide in Hokkaido District, Japan. *American Journal of Forensic Medicine and Pathology* 7(2): 104–6.

Shorter, Edward. 1975. *The making of the modern family.* New York: Basic Books.

Simonds, Wendy and Katz Rothman, Barbara. 1992. *Centuries of solace: Expressions of maternal grief in popular literature.* Philadelphia: Temple University Press.

Sirbu, Valeriu. 2008. Ritual inhumations and 'deposits' of children among the Geto-Dacians. In *Deviant burial* ed. E. M. Murphy, 71–90. Oxford: Oxbow Books.

Slater, Peter Gregg. 1977. *Children in the New England mind.* Connecticut: Archon Books.

Smith, Daniel Scott. 1985. Child-naming practices, kinship ties, and change in family attitudes in Hingham, Massachusetts, 1641 to 1880. *Journal of Social History* 18(4): 541–566.

Smart, Laura, S. 1993. Parental bereavement in Anglo American history. *OMEGA* 28(1): 49–61.

Smith, William Robertson. 1903. *Kinship and marriage in Early Arabia.* London: Adam & Charles Block.

Smith-Spark, Laura and Magnay, Diana. 2014. Belgium: Lawmakers vote for children's 'right to die' euthanasia law. *CNN.*

Stager, Lawrence and Samuel. R. Wolff. 1984. Child sacrifice in Carthage: Religious rite or population control? *Journal of Biblical Archeological Review* January: 31–46.

Stone, L. 1977. *The family, sex and marriage in England 1500–1800.* London:

Sundin, Jan. 1996. Child mortality and causes of death in a Swedish city, 1750–1869. *Historical Methods* 29(3): 93–106.

Suzman, Susan M. 1994. Names as pointers: Zulu personal naming practices. *Language in Society* 23(2): 253–272.

Suzuki, Hikaru. 2003. McFunerals: The transition of Japanese funerary services. *Asian Anthropology* 2(1): 49–78.

Tarassov, L.M. 1971. La double statuette pale'olithique de Gagarino. *Quartar* 22: 157–163.

Taylor, Alison. 2008. Aspects of deviant burial in Roman Britain. In *Deviant burial* ed. E. M. Murphy, 91–114. Oxford: Oxbow Books.

Taylor, Lou. 2010. *Mourning dress: A costume and social history*. Abingdon, Oxon, England: Routledge.

Teelucksingh, Jerome. 2006. The 'invisible child' in British West Indian slavery. *Slavery and Abolition* 27(2): 237–250.

Thomas, Aline, Chambon, Philippe, Murail, Pascal. 2011. Unpacking burial and rank: The role of children in the first monumental cemeteries of Western Europe (4600–4300 BC). *Antiquity* 85 (329).

Tsaliki, Anastasia. 2008. Unusual burials and necrophobia: An insight into the burial archaeology of fear. In *Deviant burial* ed. E. M. Murphy, 1–16. Oxford: Oxbow Books.

Ucko, Peter. 1969. Ethnography and archaeological interpretation of funerary remains. *World Archaeology* 1: 262–280.

United Nations Inter-agency Group for Child Mortality Estimation. 2011. *Levels & trends in child mortality.* United Nations Children's Fund: New York. http://www.childinfo.org/files/Child_Mortality_Report_2011.pdf

Van Setten, Hank. 1999. Album angels: Parent-child relations as reflected in 19th-century photos, made after the death of a child. *The Journal of Psychohistory* 26(4): 819–834.

Volavkova, Hana, Vaclav Havel, Chaim Potok, and United States Holocaust Memorial Museum. 1994. *I never saw another butterfly: Children's drawings and poems from the Terezin concentration camp, 1942–1944.* New York: Schocken.

Vovelle, Michelle. 1980. A century and one-half of American epitaphs (1660–1813): Toward the study of collective attitudes about death. *Comparative Studies in Society and History* 22(4): 534–547.

Vreeland, James, M. and Aiden Cockburn. 1980. Mummies of Peru In *Mummies, disease,* eds. A. Cockburn, E. Cockburn, and T.A. Reyman, 154–189. Cambridge University Press.

Weiss-Krejci, Estella. 2008. The unusual life, unusual death and the fate of the corpse: A case study from dynastic Europe. In *Deviant burial* ed. E. M. Murphy, 169–190. Oxford: Oxbow Books.

Westermarck, Edward. 1968. *A short history of marriage.* NY: Humanities Press.

Williamson, L. 1978. Infanticide: An anthropological analysis. In *Infanticide and the value,* ed. M. Kohl, 61–75. Buffalo, N.Y.: Prometheus Books.

Wilson, S. (1984). The myth of motherhood: The historical view of European child-rearing. *Social History* 9(2): 181–198.

Wood, Charles H., Magno de Carvalho, Jose Alberto, and Guimaraes Horta, Claudia Julia. 2010. The color of child mortality in Brazil, 1950–2000: Social progress and persistent racial inequality. *Latin American Research Review* 45(2): 115–139.

World Bank. 2014. *Indigenous peoples overview.* http://www.worldbank.org/en/topic/indigenous peoples/overview

World Health Organization. 2013. *WHO- Children: Reducing Mortality.* http://www.who.int/mediacentre/factsheets/fs178/en/

Zagorska, Ilga. 2008. The use of ochre in stone age burials of the East Baltic. *BAR International Series* 1768: 115.

Index

C

F

G

L

M

N

O

P

Q

R

S

T

U

V

W

X

Y

Z